AF213855

Studies in Computational Intelligence

Volume 1131

Series Editor

Janusz Kacprzyk, Polish Academy of Sciences, Warsaw, Poland

The series "Studies in Computational Intelligence" (SCI) publishes new developments and advances in the various areas of computational intelligence—quickly and with a high quality. The intent is to cover the theory, applications, and design methods of computational intelligence, as embedded in the fields of engineering, computer science, physics and life sciences, as well as the methodologies behind them. The series contains monographs, lecture notes and edited volumes in computational intelligence spanning the areas of neural networks, connectionist systems, genetic algorithms, evolutionary computation, artificial intelligence, cellular automata, self-organizing systems, soft computing, fuzzy systems, and hybrid intelligent systems. Of particular value to both the contributors and the readership are the short publication timeframe and the world-wide distribution, which enable both wide and rapid dissemination of research output.

Indexed by SCOPUS, DBLP, WTI Frankfurt eG, zbMATH, SCImago.

All books published in the series are submitted for consideration in Web of Science.

Loveleen Gaur · Ajith Abraham · Reuel Ajith
Editors

AI and Neuro-Degenerative Diseases

Insights and Solutions

Springer

Editors
Loveleen Gaur
Amity International Business School
Amity University
Noida, India

Ajith Abraham
Bennett University
Greater Noida, India

Reuel Ajith
Ameos Klinikum St Clemens
Oberhausen, North Rhine-Westphalia
Germany

ISSN 1860-949X ISSN 1860-9503 (electronic)
Studies in Computational Intelligence
ISBN 978-3-031-53147-7 ISBN 978-3-031-53148-4 (eBook)
https://doi.org/10.1007/978-3-031-53148-4

© The Editor(s) (if applicable) and The Author(s), under exclusive license to Springer Nature Switzerland AG 2024

This work is subject to copyright. All rights are solely and exclusively licensed by the Publisher, whether the whole or part of the material is concerned, specifically the rights of translation, reprinting, reuse of illustrations, recitation, broadcasting, reproduction on microfilms or in any other physical way, and transmission or information storage and retrieval, electronic adaptation, computer software, or by similar or dissimilar methodology now known or hereafter developed.
The use of general descriptive names, registered names, trademarks, service marks, etc. in this publication does not imply, even in the absence of a specific statement, that such names are exempt from the relevant protective laws and regulations and therefore free for general use.
The publisher, the authors and the editors are safe to assume that the advice and information in this book are believed to be true and accurate at the date of publication. Neither the publisher nor the authors or the editors give a warranty, expressed or implied, with respect to the material contained herein or for any errors or omissions that may have been made. The publisher remains neutral with regard to jurisdictional claims in published maps and institutional affiliations.

This Springer imprint is published by the registered company Springer Nature Switzerland AG
The registered company address is: Gewerbestrasse 11, 6330 Cham, Switzerland

Paper in this product is recyclable.

Contents

Demystifying the Role of Artificial Intelligence in Neurodegenerative Diseases

Sandeep Mathur and Aditi Jaiswal

Abstract In recent years, older people are increasingly diagnosed with neurodegenerative disorders. Artificial Intelligence (AI) algorithms can aid in early detection and accurate diagnosis of these diseases, enabling timely interventions and personalized treatment plans. These algorithms also predict disease progression and prognosis, providing valuable insights into disease trajectories and clinical decision-making. AI-powered image processing techniques detect subtle structural and functional changes in the brain, aiding in the identification of disease-specific biomarkers. These biomarkers facilitate early intervention and provide objective measures of treatment efficacy, essential for clinical trials and drug development. However, challenges remain in applying AI to neurodegenerative diseases, such as data privacy, security, and integrating AI tools into routine clinical practice. AI has immense potential to transform our understanding of, detection, and treatment of neurodegenerative illnesses, contributing significantly to the development of effective therapies and improved patient care.

Keywords Neurodegenerative diseases · Artificial Intelligence · Biomarkers · Neuroimaging · Progression

1 Introduction

A significant global health issue is the prevalence of neurodegenerative disorders like ALS, Parkinson's disease, and Alzheimer's disease. In recent years, the development of AI has given rise to fresh optimism in the study of neurodegenerative diseases. AI techniques enable the integration and analysis of diverse datasets, such as clinical records, genetic information, neuroimaging scans, and molecular profiles. AI algorithms can assist in early detection by analyzing various data sources, facilitating the identification of subtle disease markers or prodromal symptoms that may precede clinical manifestations. AI-powered diagnostic models can enhance the accuracy and

S. Mathur (✉) · A. Jaiswal
Noida International University, Greater Noida, Uttar Pradesh, India
e-mail: sandeep2809@gmail.com

© The Author(s), under exclusive license to Springer Nature Switzerland AG 2024

L. Gaur et al. (eds.), *AI and Neuro-Degenerative Diseases*, Studies in Computational Intelligence 1131, https://doi.org/10.1007/978-3-031-53148-4_1

efficiency of disease identification, aiding clinicians in making more informed decisions [1]. AI-based predictive modeling has shown promise in estimating disease progression and prognosis. AI algorithms can generate predictive models that estimate the trajectory of neurodegenerative diseases, enabling better treatment planning and resource allocation. AI-powered image processing algorithms can analyze complex neuroimaging data, identify disease-specific patterns or structural changes in the brain, and assist in accurate diagnosis and monitoring of disease progression [2]. AI-based algorithms can rapidly analyze large-scale biomedical datasets, predict drug-target interactions, and identify potential therapeutic compounds, accelerating the process of identifying promising drug candidates and designing more efficient clinical trials. AI has the potential to improve the lives of individuals affected by neurodegenerative disease and bring us closer to effective treatments and preventive strategies. The current study advises a complete, in-depth investigation of existing artificial intelligence's ability to aid in the diagnosis and analysis of major neurodegenerative disorders with the help of Brain MRI-based AI. While other different neurodegenerative disorders may exist, we will focus on Alzheimer's disease because it is the most common and symbolic of the neurodegenerative range. Alzheimer's disease (AD) is a devastating and insidious neurological illness that affects millions of people worldwide. By revealing hidden patterns and linkages inside complicated data, Data science, and artificial intelligence have the potential to completely change our knowledge of AD. AI algorithms have proven to be capable of analyzing a variety of datasets, including genetic data, neuroimaging scans, and medical records, to spot subtle illness indicators and help with early diagnosis. Early detection of AD can enable therapies like lifestyle changes and prospective medicines in the future, increasing patient outcomes and quality of life. By revealing hidden patterns and linkages inside complicated data, AI has the potential to fundamentally alter our knowledge of AD [3]. Huge datasets may be integrated and analyzed using AI algorithms, which can then explore complex relationships between genetic variants, biomarkers, cognitive tests, and clinical outcomes. Another crucial area where AI might significantly impact AD is in neuroimaging analysis. To make an accurate diagnosis, track the development of the disease, and forecast treatment outcomes, AI systems can analyze complicated pictures, spot tiny anomalies, and extract quantitative characteristics. Virtual screening and predictive modeling are two AI-based techniques that can analyze and predict interactions between drugs and their targets while also making it easier to find possible therapeutic molecules [4]. AI has the potential to completely transform AD diagnosis, treatment, and management, providing previously unheard-of chances to understand the complexity of this fatal illness and improve the quality of life for AD patients and their families while reducing the risk of death.

2 Literature Review

Table 1 focuses on the advancements in the diagnosis and treatment of neurodegenerative diseases using Artificial Intelligence.

3 The Transformative Role of AI in Healthcare

AI has become a game changer in healthcare, revolutionizing disease detection and management. By leveraging AI algorithms and techniques, healthcare professionals can harness the power of big data sets, advanced imaging technology, and advanced analytics to improve patient outcomes. This article provides an in-depth exploration of how AI is used in healthcare, with a particular focus on its application in disease detection, diagnosis, and management (Fig. 1).

3.1 AI in Disease Detection

AI plays a central role in disease detection, enabling early identification and diagnosis of various conditions. Machine learning algorithms excel at analyzing medical images, such as X-rays, magnetic resonance imaging, and computed tomography, to detect abnormalities and help radiologists interpret Accurately solve complex data. These algorithms use deep learning techniques to recognize patterns and markers, helping to detect diseases like cancer, cardiovascular disorders, and neurodegenerative diseases early. In addition to medical imaging, AI facilitates the analysis of various data sources, including electronic health records, genetic information, and lifestyle data. By integrating and analyzing this data, AI algorithms can identify patterns, risk factors, and predictive markers that help identify people at high risk for certain diseases. This early warning system enables healthcare providers to proactively intervene, initiating treatment and prevention measures promptly.

3.2 AI in Disease Diagnosis

AI algorithms make an important contribution to accurate and efficient disease diagnosis. Using machine learning techniques, AI can process large volumes of patient data, from symptoms and medical history to genetic profiles and test results. By analyzing these data sets, AI algorithms generate diagnostic insights, helping healthcare providers make more informed and informed decisions. AI-powered diagnostic tools based on natural language processing (NLP) and speech recognition facilitate the extraction and interpretation of medical information from clinical notes.

Table 1 Reviewing multiple authors' previous research work

Sno	Experiment	Author	Outcome	Future direction	References
1	"Applications of AI in Healthcare: A review"	"Mohammed Yousef Shaheen"	AI revolutionizes healthcare by automating research, and clinical studies, and addressing inequitable access	AI and ML advancements in healthcare improve patient care and efficiency	[1]
2	"Artificial intelligence in neurodegenerative diseases: A review of available tools with a focus on Machine Learning techniques"	"Alexandra-Maria Tăuţan, Bogdan Ionescu, Emiliano Santarnecchi"	Computational methods are increasingly used to monitor and diagnose neurodegenerative illnesses like ALS, MSA, PD, and AD	Improved early neurodegenerative disease detection using biomarkers, memory testing, and integrative strategies	[2]
3	"Multi-Layer Picture of Neurodegenerative Diseases: Lessons from the Use of Big Data through Artificial Intelligence"	"Andrea Termine, Carlo Fabrizio, Claudia Strafella, Valerio Caputo, Laura Petrosini, Carlo Caltagirone, Emiliano Giardina, and Raffaella Cascella"	Deep learning enhances understanding of neurodegenerative illnesses using biomedical data integration for precision medicine	AI analyzes biomedical data for precision medicine, targeting therapeutic targets	[3]

(continued)

Table 1 (continued)

Sno	Experiment	Author	Outcome	Future direction	References
4	"Internet of Things (IoT) and PKI based Security Architecture"	"Sandeep Mathur, Ankita Arora"	IoT revolutionizes sectors by connecting physical devices, enhancing efficiency, customer service, and productivity	IoT is expected to significantly impact businesses, improving productivity, customer service, decision-making, and cost-effectiveness through wireless innovations and real-time data exchange	[4]
5	"Artificial Intelligence on FDG PET Images Identifies Mild Cognitive Impairment Patients with Neurodegenerative Disease"	"Joan Prats-Climent, Maria Teresa Gandia-Ferrero, Irene Torres-Espallardo, Lourdes Álvarez-Sanchez, Begoña Martínez-Sanchis, Consuelo Cháfer-Pericás, Ignacio Gómez-Rico, Leonor Cerdá-Alberich, Fernando Aparici-Robles, Miquel Baquero-Toledo, María José Rodríguez-Álvarez, Luis Martí-Bonmatí"	PDT algorithm validated for MCI patients, identifying neurodegenerative illnesses with 79% precision, 88% sensibility, and 71% specificity	3D neural network model detects neurodegenerative diseases in MCI patients	[5]
6	"Data science in neurodegenerative disease: its capabilities, limitations, and perspectives"	"Sepehr Golriz Khatami, Sarah Mubeen, Martin Hofmann-Apitius"	Computational models and artificial intelligence enhance neurodegenerative disease research	Clinical data constraints hinder neurodegeneration studies; machine learning and AI techniques offer potential solutions	[6]
7	"Artificial Intelligence for Alzheimer's Disease: Promise or Challenge?"	"Carlo Fabrizio, Andrea Termine, Carlo Caltagirone, Giulia Sancesario"	AI advances AD research through data sharing and big data analysis	AI advances AD research, but challenges require objective assessment	[7]

(continued)

Table 1 (continued)

Sno	Experiment	Author	Outcome	Future direction	References
8	"Artificial intelligence and neuropsychological measures: The case of Alzheimer's disease"	"Petronilla Battista, Christian Salvatore, Manuela Berlingeri, Antonio Cerasa, Isabella Castiglioni"	Machine learning improves classification accuracy for MCI patients, predicting AD risk	Early AD impairment was identified using ML and neuropsychological testing; no research comparing accuracy	[8]
9	"Use of artificial intelligence in Alzheimer's disease detection"	"Mark Melchionna"	AI algorithms aid in AD detection in clinical settings through image processing and feature extraction	AI advances in image-based diagnosis, disease detection, and risk management	[9]
10	"Application of Artificial Intelligence techniques for the detection of Alzheimer's disease using structural MRI images"	"Xinxing Zhao, Candice Ke En Ang, U. Rajendra Acharya, Kang Hao Cheong"	AI-based CAD techniques identify early AD phases, focusing on structural MRI	Early detection and diagnosis of AD using cloud computing and smart home products	[10]

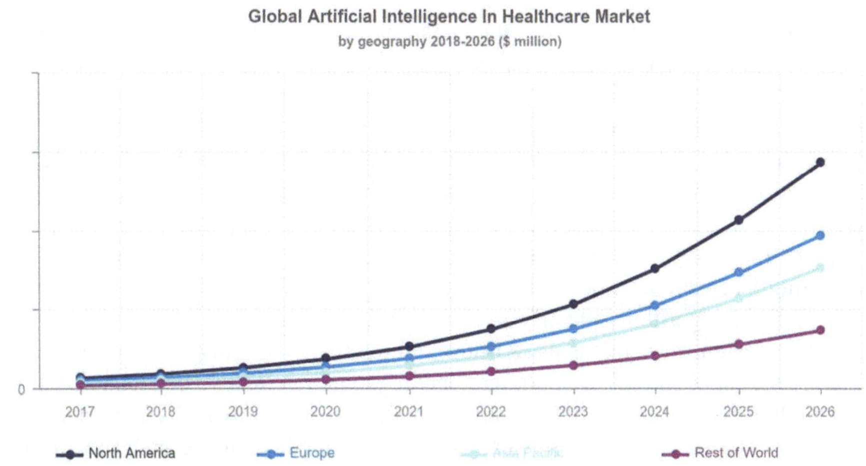

Fig.1 Graph showing AI in the healthcare market during the forecast period (2018–2026). Reprinted from "Applications of Artificial Intelligence (AI) in Healthcare" by Shaheen [1]

and interactions between patients and doctors. These tools automate the encoding, duplication, and medical documentation process, reducing administrative burdens and improving diagnostic accuracy and efficiency. In specific pathological fields, AI demonstrates outstanding capabilities. In the case of cancer, for example, AI algorithms can analyze genomic data to identify specific mutations and biomarkers, allowing for personalized treatment planning tailored to each patient. In dermatology, AI-powered systems can analyze images of skin lesions, assisting in the diagnosis of skin cancer and other dermatological conditions.

3.3 *AI in Disease Management*

The impact of AI on disease management is multifaceted, improving treatment efficiency, patient monitoring, and personalized care planning. Using predictive analytics, AI algorithms can assess disease progression, treatment response, and potential complications, allowing healthcare providers to tailor interventions for each patient. This personalized approach optimizes treatment results while minimizing side effects. Remote patient monitoring powered by AI and Internet of Things (IoT) devices enables continuous monitoring of a patient's vital signs, activity levels, and medication adherence. AI algorithms analyze this data in real time, alerting healthcare providers to any discrepancies or potential health risks. This proactive monitoring improves patient safety, facilitates early intervention, and reduces readmissions. In the area of chronic diseases, such as diabetes or cardiovascular disease [5]. AI algorithms help develop personalized care plans that take into account a person's risk factors, comorbidities, and lifestyle factors. each individual. These plans may include medication recommendations, diet, and exercise advice, promote self-management, and improve patient outcomes. AI is also revolutionizing surgical procedures, with robot-assisted surgeries growing in popularity. Surgical robots, guided by AI algorithms, improve accuracy, visualization, and dexterity, reduce human error and improve surgical outcomes. AI algorithms can analyze surgical data to optimize surgical techniques, reduce complications, and improve overall patient safety.

Drug discovery and development benefit greatly from AI capabilities. By analyzing large amounts of scientific literature, and genomic and molecular structure data, AI algorithms identify potential drugs, predict their effectiveness, and facilitate design. new therapies. AI-powered simulations help predict drug-target interactions and optimize drug dosages, leading to more effective treatments. Artificial intelligence has changed the healthcare industry, especially in disease detection, diagnosis, and management. From early detection to medical image analysis to accurate diagnosis based on patient data, AI algorithms have proven unsurpassed ability to improve patient outcomes. Through personalized treatment plans, remote patient monitoring, and optimized surgical procedures, AI continues to drive healthcare operations, delivering effective interventions. more efficient, effective, and personalized. The integration of AI into healthcare is revolutionizing disease detection and management, paving the way to a future that delivers better healthcare outcomes and better patient care.

4 Early Detection and Diagnosis of Neurodegenerative Diseases Using AI

Neurodegenerative diseases, such as Alzheimer's disease, Parkinson's disease, and Huntington's disease, pose significant health challenges due to their progressive nature and debilitating effect on individuals. Early detection and accurate diagnosis of these diseases are crucial for effective treatment and management. AI has become a powerful tool in the medical field, providing promising solutions for the early detection and diagnosis of neurodegenerative diseases. This article provides a comprehensive overview of how AI is being used to aid early detection and diagnosis, helping to improve patient outcomes.

4.1 Information Procurement and Preprocessing

AI-based approaches rely on large amounts of data, including medical imaging scans, genetic information, clinical records, and biomarkers. This data is collected and preprocessed to remove noise, standardize the format, and ensure compatibility between different sources. Advanced techniques, such as deep learning algorithms, are used to extract relevant characteristics and patterns from the data, allowing for more accurate analysis.

4.2 *Imaging Analysis*

Medical imaging plays an important role in the early detection and diagnosis of neurodegenerative diseases. AI algorithms, especially convolutional neural networks (CNNs), have shown outstanding performance in analyzing various imaging modalities, including magnetic resonance imaging (MRI), positron tomography emission layer (PET), and computed tomography (CT). These algorithms can detect small changes in brain structure, identify specific biomarkers, and predict disease progression with great accuracy.

4.3 *Biomarkers Identification*

Biomarkers are measurable indicators of disease-related processes or responses in the body. AI techniques, such as machine learning and deep learning, can analyze large-scale biomarker data sets to identify patterns and correlations that may indicate neurodegenerative diseases. By leveraging these models, AI models can assist in the early identification of people at high risk for these diseases, enabling proactive intervention and personalized treatment planning.

4.4 *Prescient Modeling*

AI models can integrate a variety of data sources, including clinical, genetic, and environmental factors, to develop predictive models of neurodegenerative diseases. These models use machine learning algorithms to assess an individual's risk and provide early warnings. They can also predict disease progression and response to specific treatments, allowing healthcare professionals to tailor interventions based on individual patient characteristics.

4.5 *Computerized Biomarkers and Wearable Gadgets*

Advances in wearable devices, such as smartwatches and fitness trackers, have opened up new avenues for continuous tracking of individuals. AI algorithms can analyze data collected by these devices, including sleep patterns, gait analysis, heart rate variability, and other physiological parameters, to detect subtle changes associated with related to neurodegenerative diseases. These digital biomarkers provide a non-invasive and cost-effective means of early detection and monitoring.

4.6 Decision Support Systems

AI-based decision support systems can help healthcare professionals accurately diagnose and plan treatment for neurodegenerative diseases. By analyzing patient data and comparing it with large databases, these systems can provide clinicians with evidence-based recommendations, improving diagnostic accuracy and reducing diagnostic errors. They can also help monitor disease progression and evaluate the effectiveness of treatment interventions.

Although AI holds great promise in the early detection and diagnosis of neurodegenerative diseases, several challenges need to be addressed. These include the need for diverse, high-quality data sets, regulatory considerations, ethical implications, and the importance of ensuring that AI models are transparent and explainable. Further research and collaboration are needed to refine AI techniques, validate their performance, and incorporate them into routine clinical practice. Artificial intelligence has the potential to revolutionize the early detection and diagnosis of neurodegenerative diseases, delivering better patient outcomes and personalized treatment strategies. By leveraging AI algorithms to analyze data, interpret images, identify biomarkers, and predictive models, healthcare professionals can make informed decisions and intervene at early stages, allowing for timely intervention and improved patient care. However, addressing the challenges and ensuring the ethical and responsible implementation of AI in healthcare will be critical to successfully integrating AI into routine clinical practice [6].

5 Image Analysis

AI has revolutionized the diagnosis and monitoring of neurodegenerative diseases thanks to its powerful image analysis capabilities. AI algorithms, especially Convolutional Neural Networks (CNNs), have been widely used to analyze various medical imaging modalities including Magnetic Resonance Imaging (MRI), Emission Tomography Positron (PET), and computed tomography (CT) (Fig. 2).

By harnessing AI's image analysis capabilities, healthcare professionals can benefit from increased accuracy, efficiency, and objectivity in the detection and diagnosis of neurodegenerative diseases. AI-based image analysis algorithms excel at identifying subtle changes and abnormalities in medical images that may indicate the presence or progression of neurodegenerative diseases. These algorithms can automatically analyze images, recognize patterns, and detect specific biomarkers associated with these diseases. In Alzheimer's disease, for example, AI can assess

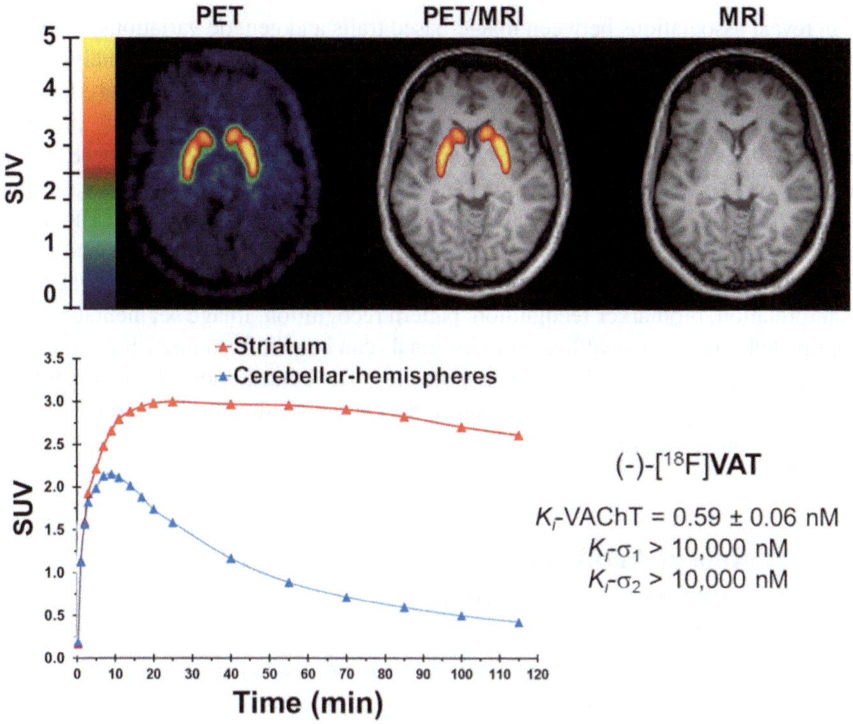

Fig. 2 PET study of (−)-[18F] VAT in a healthy human subject. PET (top left). PET/MRI (top middle) and MR (top right) images; time-activity curves (bottom) for striatum (red triangles) and cerebellar hemispheres (blue triangles). Reprinted from "Detecting neurodegenerative disease from MRI: a brief review on a deep learning perspective" by Noor et al. [10]

brain atrophy patterns and identify the presence of characteristic biomarkers, such as amyloid plaques or neurofibrillary tangles. By quantifying these biomarkers, AI can provide valuable insights into disease progression, help predict outcomes, and aid in treatment decision-making. AI algorithms master image segmentation, an important process in neural image analysis. They can accurately and automatically segment brain structures, such as the hippocampus, cortex, or subcortical regions, allowing precise measurement of volume changes and detection of abnormalities. This allows healthcare professionals to more accurately and effectively track disease progression and response to treatment. Another important application of AI in neurodegenerative diseases is the extraction of radiometric features from medical images. Radiomics involves the collection of a large number of quantitative features from images, providing detailed information about tumor characteristics or specific patterns of disease. In the context of neurodegenerative diseases, AI algorithms can analyze radiometric features extracted from neuroimaging data to identify disease-specific markers and extract information. relate to. In addition, the integration of radioactivity with genetic information, known as radiogenic genes, can reveal associations between image-based traits and genetic variations, shedding light on heterogeneity. disease and potential targets. AI-based image analysis also facilitates automatic screening and classification in the diagnosis of neurodegenerative diseases [7]. By analyzing medical images, AI algorithms can flag potential abnormalities or prioritize cases that need immediate attention. This speed up the diagnostic process, allowing healthcare professionals to focus on severe cases and deliver timely interventions to patients with neurodegenerative diseases. The image analysis capabilities of AI have greatly enhanced the field of diagnosis and monitoring of neurodegenerative diseases. By leveraging AI algorithms for medical image interpretation, biomarker recognition, pattern recognition, image segmentation, and automated screening, healthcare professionals can benefit from precision, improved efficacy, and personalized treatment strategies. The contribution of AI in the diagnosis of neurodegenerative diseases promises early detection, effective intervention, and better outcomes for patients in the future.

6 The Role of Artificial Intelligence in Drug Discovery for Neurodegenerative Diseases

Neurodegenerative diseases, such as Alzheimer's disease, Parkinson's disease, and Huntington's disease, pose significant challenges in terms of treatment development due to their complex nature and limited understanding of the underlying mechanisms. copy. However, AI has emerged as a powerful tool in the field of drug discovery, offering promising solutions for identifying and developing effective therapies for degenerative diseases. nerve. This article provides a comprehensive overview of how AI is being used to aid drug discovery, leading to potential breakthroughs in the treatment of these debilitating conditions (Fig. 3).

6.1 *Data Mining and Analysis*

AI algorithms are capable of analyzing large-scale data sets, including genomic data, medical records, protein structures, and scientific literature. By exploring and integrating these diverse data sources, AI can identify potential drug targets, uncover disease-related pathways, and discover new biomarkers associated with diseases. neurodegenerative disease. This data-driven approach provides researchers with valuable insights and guidance in the selection of promising therapeutic candidates.

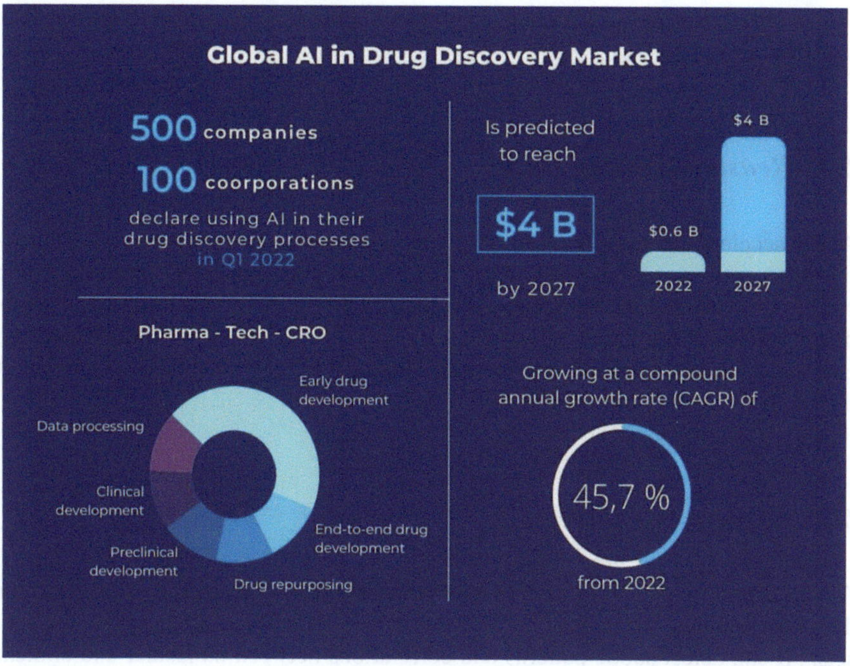

Fig. 3 AI for drug discovery and development market is expected to reach $4,815 million by 2027. Reprinted from "Neurodegenerative diseases and oxidative stress" by Barnham et al. [11]

6.2 Predictive Model

AI techniques, such as machine learning and deep learning, enable the development of predictive models for drug discovery. These models use sophisticated algorithms to analyze and interpret biological data, predict drug-target interactions, evaluate compound properties, and estimate potential toxicity. By simulating and predicting the efficacy of drug candidates, AI helps researchers prioritize the most promising compounds for further development, reducing the time and resources required for testing.

6.3 Virtual Screening and Drug Design

AI plays an important role in virtual screening and computer-aided drug design. By leveraging AI algorithms, researchers can virtually sift through large libraries of compounds and identify molecules with potential therapeutic activity against specific targets or pathways involved. to neurodegenerative diseases. In addition, AI techniques, such as generalization modeling and reinforcement learning, facilitate the generation of new chemical structures with desired properties, allowing for the design of candidates. The drug is optimized to increase effectiveness and reduce side effects.

6.4 Reusing Existing Drugs

AI can accelerate drug reuse by analyzing large-scale data sets and identifying potential therapeutic uses for existing drugs. By leveraging AI algorithms, researchers can predict new indications for approved drugs, enabling rapid development of treatments for neurodegenerative diseases. This approach offers the advantage of using existing safety and toxicity data, thereby reducing the costs and time associated with traditional drug development.

6.5 Explore Biomarkers

AI algorithms help identify disease-specific biomarkers that can serve as targets for drug development and indicators of treatment response. By analyzing complex data sets, AI can detect subtle patterns and correlations between molecular and clinical data, leading to the discovery of new biomarkers that reflect disease progression, response to treatment, and patient stratification. AI biomarker discovery enables the development of personalized therapies and facilitates the assessment of treatment efficacy in clinical trials.

6.6 Clinical Trial Optimization

AI techniques optimize clinical trial design and accelerate the evaluation of potential drugs. AI algorithms can analyze patient data, identify relevant subpopulations, and predict patient responses to specific treatments. This information allows for more efficient trial recruitment, better trial design, and better patient stratification, leading to higher success rates and lower costs in clinical trials for these diseases neurodegeneration.

6.7 Collaboration and Knowledge Sharing

AI facilitates collaboration and knowledge sharing between researchers and pharmaceutical companies. AI platforms and databases enable the integration and sharing of data, models, and information, fostering a collaborative environment for drug discovery. This collective intelligence improves the efficiency and effectiveness of research efforts, accelerates discoveries, and fosters interdisciplinary collaboration in the field of drug development against neurodegenerative diseases. The process of finding new drugs to treat neurodegenerative disorders may be completely transformed by artificial intelligence. Researchers can find and create novel therapeutics with enhanced efficacy and shorter development times by utilizing AI algorithms for data mining, predictive modeling, virtual screening, drug repurposing, biomarker discovery, clinical trial optimization, and cooperation [8]. AI's contributions to drug development raise the possibility of developing viable therapeutics for neurodegenerative illnesses and enhancing the lives of millions of those affected globally.

7 Personalized Medicine for Patients with Neurodegenerative Diseases

AI plays a central role in advancing personalized medicine for patients with neurodegenerative diseases. By harnessing the capabilities of AI, healthcare professionals can tailor treatments and interventions to individual patients based on their unique characteristics and disease progression. Below is a detailed exploration of AI's contribution to personalized medicine in the context of neurodegenerative diseases:

7.1 Risk Assessment and Prediction Model

AI algorithms can analyze a variety of patient data, including medical records, genetic information, lifestyle factors, and biomarker profiles to develop predictive models. These models assess an individual's risk of developing neurodegenerative diseases and predict disease progression. By identifying high-risk individuals at an early stage, healthcare professionals can implement prevention and intervention measures to delay or reduce the onset of the disease.

7.2 Accurate Diagnosis

AI-based diagnostic models rely on machine learning algorithms to interpret complex patient data, including medical imaging scans, genetic variants, and clinical symptoms. By integrating these data sources, AI can improve diagnostic accuracy and speed, helping to more accurately identify neurodegenerative diseases. This allows for early intervention and treatment planning tailored to the specific condition of each patient.

7.3 Prognosis of Response to Treatment

AI algorithms analyze patient data to predict individual responses to different treatment options. By considering factors such as genetics, biomarker profiles, and clinical characteristics, AI models can help healthcare professionals select the most effective treatment strategies for each disease. core. This personalized approach improves treatment outcomes and minimizes potential side effects by optimizing drug dosing, therapy selection, and monitoring procedures.

7.4 Drug Selection and Optimization

AI facilitates personalized medicine by assisting in the selection and optimization of drugs for neurodegenerative diseases. By analyzing patient-specific genetic information and biomarker profiles, AI algorithms can predict individual drug responses, identify potential side effects, and guide drug selection. unify. AI-based computer models can also optimize drug dosages and treatment regimens, ensuring maximum efficacy and safety for every patient.

7.5 Continuous Monitoring and Remote Care

Wearable devices and digital health technology, combined with AI algorithms, enable continuous monitoring of patients with neurodegenerative diseases. AI-powered systems can analyze real-time data from wearables, such as smartwatches and activity trackers, for early detection of signs of disease progression, assessment, and evaluation. motor function, monitor vital signs, and assess medication adherence. This remote monitoring allows for personalized care and rapid intervention, even outside of traditional healthcare settings.

7.6 Treatment Adjustment and Decision Support

AI-based decision support systems provide healthcare professionals with evidence-based recommendations for treatment adjustment and monitoring. By analyzing patient data, including clinical records, biomarker trends, and real-time sensor data, the AI algorithm can recommend treatment plan adjustments based on each individual's response. individual and disease progression. This personalized decision support helps healthcare professionals make informed choices, optimize treatment outcomes, and improve patient care.

7.7 *Patient Empowerment and Education*

AI-powered tools and applications empower patients by providing personalized information, educational resources, and self-management support. Virtual assistants and mobile apps can provide personalized information, medication adherence reminders, lifestyle recommendations, and access to support communities. These AI-powered tools improve patient engagement, self-care, and overall health for people with neurodegenerative diseases.

The integration of AI in personalized medicine is revolutionizing the approach to neurodegenerative diseases. By leveraging AI algorithms for predictive modeling, accurate diagnosis, prediction of treatment response, drug selection, continuous monitoring, treatment adjustment, and patient empowerment, Healthcare professionals can provide tailored care and improve outcomes for patients with neurodegenerative diseases. AI-based personalized medicine holds the promise of optimizing treatment strategies, improving patients' quality of life, and ultimately advancing the field of neurodegenerative disease management.

8 Controlling Diseases Progression and Prediction

AI plays an important role in controlling disease progression and predicting neurodegenerative diseases. By leveraging AI capabilities, healthcare professionals can gain valuable insights into disease trajectories, predict disease progression, and implement proactive interventions. Here's an in-depth exploration of how AI helps control disease progression and predict neurodegenerative diseases (Fig. 4):

8.1 *Disease Progression Pattern*

AI algorithms analyze patient data longitudinally, including clinical records, medical imaging scans, genetic information, and biomarker profiles to model disease progression. By identifying patterns and correlations in these data sets, AI can generate predictive models that estimate disease progression rates, identify milestones, and predict the progression of diseases. neurodegeneration. These models enable healthcare professionals to develop personalized treatment plans, monitor disease progression, and intervene at appropriate stages.

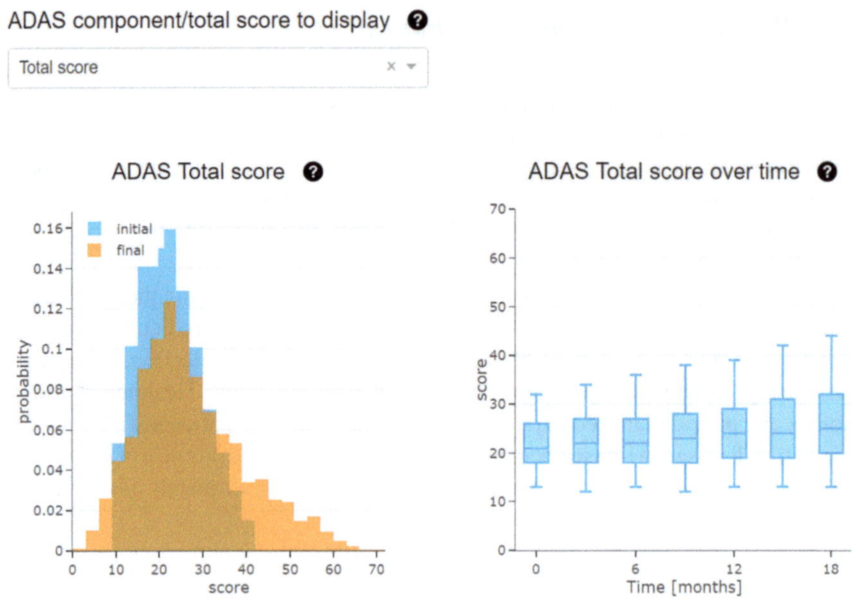

Fig. 4 Graph showing uses of AI for predicting Alzheimer's progression. Reprinted from "Application of Artificial Intelligence techniques for the detection of Alzheimer's disease using structural MRI images" by Zhao et al. [9]

8.2 Early Detection and Risk Assessment

AI algorithms analyze a variety of patient data, such as genetic variants, biomarker profiles, and lifestyle factors, to assess a person's risk of neurodegenerative diseases individual. By identifying high-risk individuals at an early stage, AI facilitates early detection and enables proactive interventions to delay or minimize disease onset. This personalized risk assessment helps implement preventive measures, make lifestyle adjustments, and target people at risk.

8.3 Prognosis of Response to Treatment

AI algorithms analyze patient-specific data, including genetics, biomarker profiles, and clinical characteristics, to predict individual responses to different treatment options. By considering these factors, AI models can help healthcare professionals choose the most effective treatment strategies for each patient. This personalized approach improves treatment outcomes by optimizing drug dosage, therapy selection, and monitoring procedures based on individual responses.

8.4 Adaptive Treatment Strategies

AI-based decision support systems can analyze patient data in real time, continuously monitor disease progression, and adjust treatment strategies accordingly. By integrating data from wearables, sensors, and electronic health records, AI algorithms can detect changes in disease status, assess treatment effectiveness, and recommend adjustments to the treatment plan. treatment plan. These adaptive strategies ensure that interventions are tailored to the changing needs of patients with neurodegenerative diseases.

8.5 Prognostic Tool

AI algorithms can analyze large-scale data sets to develop prognostic tools that help predict disease outcomes and patient prognosis. By integrating a variety of data sources, such as clinical records, imaging data, and biomarkers, AI can identify prognostic markers and risk factors associated with progression. of disease. These tools enable healthcare professionals to estimate disease trajectories, predict complications, and make informed decisions about patient care and treatment options.

8.6 Personal Disease Management

AI-powered platforms and applications enable patients to provide personalized disease management tools. These tools, such as virtual assistants and mobile apps, can offer medication reminders, symptom tracking, lifestyle recommendations, and access to support communities. Using AI algorithms, these platforms adapt to individual needs, improving personalized care, patient engagement, and overall disease management. Integrating AI into disease progression monitoring and prediction of neurodegenerative diseases offers significant benefits. By leveraging AI algorithms for disease progression modeling, early detection, treatment response prediction, adaptive treatment strategies, prognostic tools, and personalized disease management, professionals can optimize patient care, stage interventions at the right stage, and improve patient outcomes. AI-based approaches hold promise to advance the understanding and management of neurodegenerative diseases, thereby improving patients' quality of life.

9 Remote Monitoring and Supporting Tools for Healthcare Providers

AI plays an important role in managing the monitoring and care of patients with neurodegenerative diseases remotely and provides tools to support healthcare providers. Strong. By leveraging AI capabilities, remote monitoring becomes more efficient, allowing healthcare providers to monitor patient's condition, deliver timely interventions and improve overall patient care. Here's an in-depth exploration of how AI manages telemedicine and monitoring, as well as supporting tools for healthcare providers in the context of neurodegenerative diseases:

9.1 Remote Patient Monitoring

AI, combined with wearable devices and remote sensors, enables continuous remote monitoring of patients with neurodegenerative diseases. These devices collect real-time data on vital signs, activity levels, sleep patterns, and other physiological parameters. AI algorithms can analyze this data, detect abnormalities or changes in a patient's health, and alert healthcare providers to potential problems. This remote monitoring enables early detection of symptoms, prompt intervention, and optimal disease management.

9.2 Predictive Analytics

AI algorithms mine patient data, including historical records, genetic information, and biomarker profiles, to develop predictive models. These models can predict disease progression, identify potential complications, and estimate future healthcare needs. Using AI-driven predictive analytics, healthcare providers can proactively plan and allocate resources, delivering personalized and optimized interventions. improve patient care.

9.3 Remote and Virtual Consultation

Artificial intelligence technologies enable telemedicine and virtual consultations, facilitating remote communication between healthcare providers and patients. AI-powered chatbots or virtual assistants can help patients manage their condition, answer basic medical questions, and provide educational resources. This reduces the burden on healthcare providers and allows rapid access to medical advice and support for patients with neurodegenerative diseases, regardless of their geographic location.

9.4 Decision Support System

AI-based decision support systems provide healthcare providers with evidence-based treatment recommendations and guidelines. By analyzing patient data and comparing it with large databases, AI algorithms can help healthcare providers make informed decisions about diagnosis, treatment planning, and management. medicine for patients with neurodegenerative diseases. These systems improve diagnostic accuracy, support personalized treatment strategies, and reduce the risk of medical errors.

9.5 Data Analysis and Clinical Insights

AI algorithms can analyze large-scale datasets, including electronic health records, medical image scans, and clinical notes, to derive valuable insights. By integrating and analyzing these data sources, AI can identify patterns, correlations, and trends in patient data, empowering healthcare providers with insights. Clinicians can guide treatment decisions, optimize care plans, and identify potential research opportunities in the field of neurodegenerative diseases.

9.6 Care Coordination and Patient Management

AI-powered platforms and applications facilitate coordinated care and patient management for people with neurodegenerative diseases. These tools streamline communication between healthcare providers, caregivers, and patients, enabling seamless information sharing, appointment booking, and medication reminders. AI-powered care management platforms improve patient engagement, reduce treatment gaps, and improve coordination within the multidisciplinary care team.

AI is managing the remote monitoring and care of neurodegenerative diseases through remote patient monitoring, predictive analytics, telemedicine, decision support systems, analytical data analysis, and a care coordination platform. These AI-powered tools improve the quality of care, enable rapid intervention, and improve patient outcomes. In addition, supporting tools for healthcare providers, such as AI-based decision support systems, data analytics platforms, and care coordination tools, help Healthcare professionals make informed decisions, optimize patient care, and manage complex neurodegenerative disease cases. The integration of AI into remote monitoring and care offers promising advances in providing personalized and efficient healthcare for patients with neurodegenerative diseases.

10 Artificial Intelligence in Alzheimer's Disease

AI plays a crucial role in finding Alzheimer's disease, addressing the need for early detection and accurate diagnosis, as well as providing insights into disease progression and personalized treatment strategies. Alzheimer's disease, a progressive neurodegenerative condition, poses significant challenges due to its complex nature and subtle initial symptoms. AI offers several advantages in this context. AI algorithms can analyze vast amounts of medical data, including neuroimaging scans, genetic information, cognitive assessments, and clinical records. By processing and integrating these diverse data sources, AI algorithms can identify patterns and biomarkers associated with Alzheimer's disease. This enables the detection of subtle changes in the brain, such as atrophy in specific regions or the presence of amyloid plaques and tau tangles, even before noticeable symptoms manifest. Early detection is crucial as it allows for timely interventions, access to potential disease-modifying treatments, and the ability to plan for future care needs. AI-based image analysis is instrumental in the diagnosis of Alzheimer's disease. Neuroimaging techniques, such as MRI and PET scans, provide valuable information about brain structure and function. However, interpreting these complex images can be challenging for healthcare professionals. AI algorithms, particularly those utilizing deep learning, excel at analyzing these images, accurately detecting abnormalities, and assisting in the diagnosis of Alzheimer's disease. This improves diagnostic accuracy and reduces the likelihood of misdiagnosis, leading to more appropriate treatment and care planning. AI enables the integration and analysis of various data types, including genetic information and clinical records. Genetic factors play a significant role in the development and progression of Alzheimer's disease. AI algorithms can analyze genetic data to identify specific risk factors, susceptibility genes, and potential treatment targets. This genetic information, combined with other clinical data, facilitates personalized medicine approaches for Alzheimer's patients. Tailoring treatment plans based on individual characteristics improves treatment efficacy and patient outcomes [9] as shown in Fig. 5.

Another critical aspect of AI in Alzheimer's disease is its ability to predict disease progression. AI models can analyze longitudinal patient data, tracking changes in cognitive function, biomarker levels, and clinical assessments over time. These predictive models help estimate the trajectory of the disease, identify patients at higher risk of rapid decline, and determine optimal timing for interventions. Such insights enable healthcare providers to develop personalized care plans, adjust medications, and provide appropriate support to patients and their families. The importance of data cannot be overstated in the context of AI for Alzheimer's disease. The availability of large, diverse datasets is crucial for training and validating AI

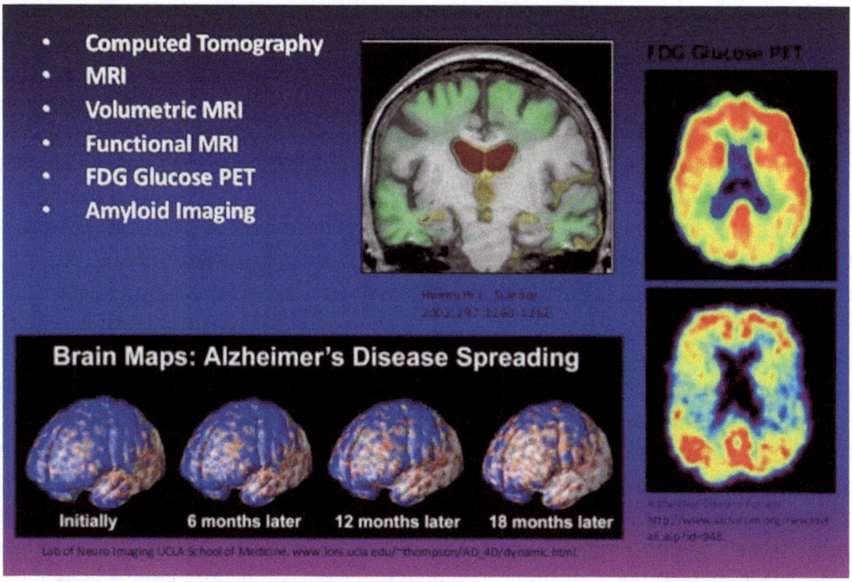

Fig. 5 Evolution of neuroimaging in Alzheimer's disease. Reprinted from "Artificial intelligence for Alzheimer's disease: promise or challenge?" by Fabrizio et al. [6]

algorithms. Organizations, research institutions, and healthcare systems are collaborating to create comprehensive databases that include clinical data, neuroimaging scans, genetic information, and cognitive assessments. These datasets serve as valuable resources for AI research and development, driving advancements in Alzheimer's detection, diagnosis, and management. AI plays a vital role in finding Alzheimer's disease by enabling early detection, accurate diagnosis, prediction of disease progression, and personalized treatment strategies. It leverages diverse data sources, including neuroimaging scans, genetic information, and clinical records, to provide valuable insights into the disease [10]. AI-powered tools and algorithms assist healthcare professionals in making informed decisions, optimizing patient care, and improving outcomes. The availability and utilization of robust datasets are critical for the advancement of AI applications in Alzheimer's disease research and clinical practice.

Several AI models can be used for diagnosing and treating Alzheimer's disease. Here are some commonly employed models:

11 Machine Learning Algorithms

AI has revolutionized the diagnosis and treatment of Alzheimer's disease by leveraging machine learning algorithms. AI algorithms analyze a variety of data, including medical imaging scans, genetic information, cognitive assessments, and biomarker profiles, to detect and diagnose Alzheimer's disease in its early stages. the beginning. Machine learning models can detect subtle patterns and changes in brain structure or function that may indicate the presence of disease. By training on large datasets, AI algorithms can learn complex patterns and relationships in the data, allowing for more accurate and efficient diagnoses. AI plays an important role in predicting disease progression and tailoring treatment strategies for patients with Alzheimer's disease. Machine learning algorithms can integrate a variety of patient data, such as demographics, genetic markers, biomarkers, and cognitive assessments, to develop predictive models [12]. These models can assess an individual's risk of developing the disease or predict disease progression. By analyzing large data sets and identifying complex patterns, AI-powered predictive models allow healthcare professionals to personalize treatment plans and track disease progression. by the time. Machine learning algorithms also help identify specific biomarkers associated with Alzheimer's disease. AI algorithms can analyze large-scale biomarker datasets, such as genetic markers, protein levels, or metabolic factors, to identify patterns and correlations that show diseases. These biomarkers can serve as diagnostic or prognostic indicators, supporting early detection and personalized treatment planning. Additionally, AI algorithms help interpret medical imaging scans, such as MRI or PET, to diagnose Alzheimer's disease. Machine learning algorithms, specifically convolutional neural networks (CNNs), can automatically analyze these images to detect brain atrophy, quantify amyloid plaque loads, or identify nerve fiber disorders terribly. By leveraging machine learning techniques [13] (Fig. 6).

AI improves the accuracy and efficiency of image interpretation, providing a valuable diagnostic aid. Machine learning algorithms also play an important role in predicting an individual's response to treatment for Alzheimer's disease. By analyzing patient data, including genetic variants, biomarker profiles, and clinical characteristics, AI models can predict how patients will respond to other treatment options. together. This personalized approach allows healthcare professionals to select the most appropriate treatment for each patient, optimizing treatment outcomes and minimizing potential side effects. The use of AI machine learning algorithms has greatly enhanced the diagnosis and treatment of Alzheimer's disease. By analyzing diverse datasets including imaging scans, biomarkers, genetic information, and clinical data, AI algorithms improve early detection, allowing treatment strategies to be tailored. personalize and help healthcare professionals more effectively care for patients with Alzheimer's disease. AI-based approaches hold promise to improve patient outcomes and accelerate research into Alzheimer's disease.

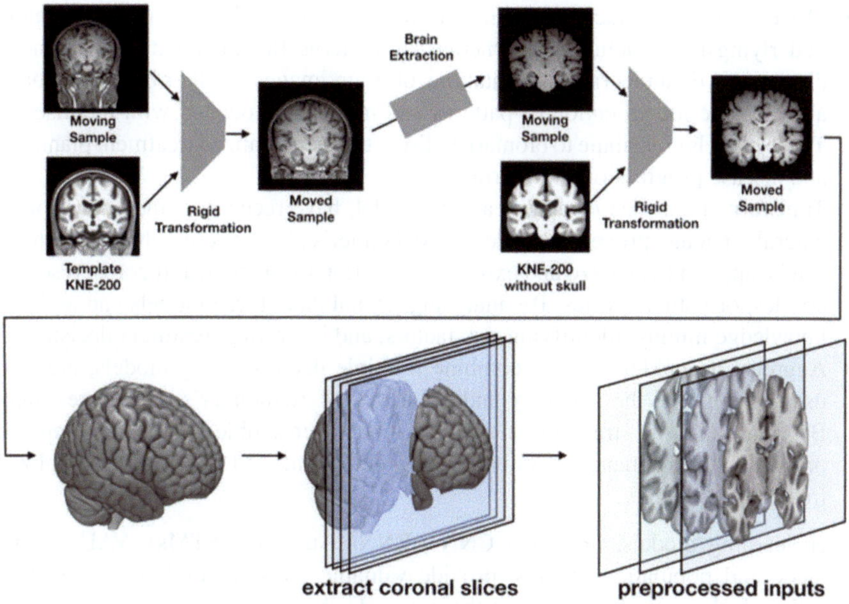

Fig. 6 Uses of convolutional neural networks (CNNs) in the identification of Alzheimer's. Reprinted from "Artificial intelligence in neurodegenerative diseases: A review of available tools with a focus on machine learning techniques" by Tăuţan et al. [2]

12 Deep Learning Models

Deep learning models have shown great promise in the field of Alzheimer's research, assisting in the detection and treatment of this disease. Several deep learning models are used to detect and treat Alzheimer's disease:

- Convolutional neural networks (CNNs) have been widely used for image analysis tasks, including medical image analysis such as MRI and PET. CNN excels at automatically extracting relevant features from brain images, enabling abnormalities, such as brain atrophy or the presence of amyloid plaques, hallmarks of Alzheimer's disease. These models improve diagnostic accuracy and facilitate early detection.
- Recurrent neural networks (RNNs), including variants such as short-term long-term memory networks (LSTMs), are used to analyze sequence data in Alzheimer's disease research. RNNs can process time series data such as cognitive assessments or biomarker measurements. By capturing time-dependent factors, these models can predict disease progression, identify subtypes of disease, and evaluate the effectiveness of interventions over time. RNNs help with personalized treatment planning and disease progression tracking.

- Model generation, such as the transform autoencoder (VAE), is used to explore underlying data structures and generate new patterns. In the context of Alzheimer's disease, VAE can learn representations of brain images or other biomarker data, allowing the identification of patterns and markers associated with the disease. These models contribute to biomarker discovery, personalized treatment planning, and disease progression monitoring.
- Transformers, a type of deep learning model, have recently gained attention in natural language processing tasks. In Alzheimer's disease research, transformers can be applied to analyze and extract information from medical records, research articles, or patient stories. By analyzing textual data, these models can assist in knowledge mining, identifying risk factors, and informing treatment decisions.
- Aggregation models, which combine multiple deep learning models, are also used to improve the accuracy and efficiency of Alzheimer's disease research. By combining the strengths of different models, ensemble models can improve prediction performance, facilitate early detection, and support personalized treatment strategies.

Deep learning models, including CNNs, RNNs (such as LSTMs), VAEs, transformers, and population models, provide valuable tools for finding and treating Alzheimer's disease. By leveraging these models, AI can improve diagnostic accuracy, predict disease progression, facilitate personalized treatment planning, and aid research efforts to understand and manage Alzheimer's disease [11]. These models have the potential to significantly impact patient care and contribute to advances in the field of Alzheimer's disease research.

13 Natural Language Processing (NLP) Models

Natural Language Processing (NLP) models have emerged as powerful tools in AI to aid in finding and treating Alzheimer's disease. These models leverage language understanding and analysis to extract valuable information from textual data. In the context of Alzheimer's research, several NLP models are commonly utilized.

- Named Entity Recognition (NER) models can automatically identify and classify disease names, medications, genes, or proteins mentioned in clinical records or research articles, facilitating knowledge extraction.
- Text classification models, including deep learning models like Convolutional Neural Networks (CNNs) or Transformers, are employed to classify text into predefined categories such as disease stage, treatment response, or risk factors.
- Sentiment analysis models can analyze patient narratives or caregiver experiences to gauge emotional well-being and quality of life.
- Topic modeling models uncover common themes discussed in research articles or patient forums, providing researchers with a deeper understanding of the disease.

- Question-answering models assist healthcare professionals by providing accurate answers to queries related to Alzheimer's diagnosis, treatment options, or caregiving strategies.
- Information extraction models extract structured data, such as biomarker values or clinical outcomes, from unstructured text, facilitating data mining and analysis. These NLP models enhance access to information, support decision-making processes, and contribute to advancing research and patient care in Alzheimer's disease.[14]

14 Generative Adversarial Networks (GANs) Models

Generative Adversarial Networks models have shown potential in the field of Alzheimer's research, offering unique capabilities for both treatment and finding approaches. While GANs are primarily known for their generative capabilities, they can be utilized in various ways in the context of Alzheimer's disease. Here are a few potential applications of GANs in treating and finding Alzheimer's using AI:

- **Synthetic Data Generation**: GANs can generate synthetic medical images, such as brain MRI scans, that closely resemble real patient data. This capability is particularly useful when the availability of labeled or diverse datasets is limited. By training GANs on existing patient data, researchers can generate additional synthetic data, increasing the sample size and diversity for training deep learning models. This enables more robust and accurate analysis, diagnosis, and treatment prediction for Alzheimer's disease.
- **Data Augmentation**: GANs can be employed to augment existing datasets for Alzheimer's research. By generating synthetic samples based on real patient data, GANs can introduce variations and simulate different disease stages, imaging perspectives, or pathological features. Augmented datasets help in training models that are more robust and generalize better to unseen data, ultimately improving the accuracy and reliability of algorithms used for diagnosing and treating Alzheimer's disease.
- **Biomarker Generation**: GANs can be used to generate synthetic biomarkers that mimic the molecular patterns associated with Alzheimer's disease. By training GANs on molecular or genetic data, they can learn the underlying distributions and generate new synthetic biomarkers. This capability aids in biomarker discovery, assisting researchers in identifying novel markers, understanding disease progression, and predicting treatment responses.
- **Disease Progression Modeling**: GANs can simulate disease progression by generating synthetic data that reflects the gradual changes observed in Alzheimer's disease. By training GANs on longitudinal patient data, they can learn the patterns of disease progression and generate new data points representing different stages of the disease. This allows for the creation of synthetic patient profiles that aid in predicting disease trajectory, planning interventions, and evaluating treatment efficacy.

- **Drug Discovery and Optimization**: GANs can generate novel drug-like molecules or optimize existing compounds for Alzheimer's treatment. By training GANs on chemical structures and their properties, they can learn the relationships between structure and activity. GANs can then generate new compounds with desired properties, aiding in the discovery of potential therapeutic candidates or optimizing existing drugs for improved efficacy and reduced side effects.

It is important to note that while GANs offer promising capabilities, their application in Alzheimer's research is still in its early stages. Further research and development are required to ensure the reliability, safety, and ethical considerations of using GANs in the diagnosis, treatment, and discovery of Alzheimer's disease [15].

15 Reinforcement Learning (Rl) Models

Reinforcement Learning (RL) models have the potential to contribute to the treatment and finding of Alzheimer's disease using AI. RL algorithms learn through trial and error interactions with an environment, aiming to maximize a reward signal. While RL is still in its early stages of application in the context of Alzheimer's disease, here are some potential areas where RL can be utilized:

- **Treatment Optimization**: RL can be employed to optimize treatment strategies for Alzheimer's disease. By formulating the treatment process as a sequential decision-making problem, RL models can learn to make optimal decisions regarding medication dosage, therapy selection, and scheduling of interventions. RL algorithms can consider patient-specific characteristics, biomarker profiles, and disease progression patterns to adapt treatments over time, optimizing the therapeutic outcomes for individuals with Alzheimer's disease.
- **Personalized Care Planning**: RL models can assist in personalized care planning for Alzheimer's patients. By considering patient data, including cognitive assessments, biomarker profiles, and lifestyle factors, RL algorithms can learn to create personalized care plans that address the unique needs and preferences of each patient. These plans can include tailored cognitive training programs, activity recommendations, and support strategies to improve overall well-being and quality of life.
- **Resource Allocation**: RL algorithms can be employed to optimize resource allocation in Alzheimer's care. With limited resources and a growing number of patients, RL models can learn to allocate resources such as healthcare professionals, diagnostic equipment, or research funding efficiently. By balancing the needs of patients and the available resources, RL can aid in improving the allocation and utilization of resources for diagnosis, treatment, and research in Alzheimer's disease.
- **Clinical Trial Design**: RL can contribute to the design of more efficient and effective clinical trials for Alzheimer's treatments. RL models can learn from previous trial data to identify optimal trial designs, including patient selection criteria,

treatment protocols, and outcome measures. By optimizing trial parameters, RL can accelerate the discovery and development of new therapies for Alzheimer's disease.

- **Decision Support Systems**: RL algorithms can be integrated into decision support systems to assist healthcare professionals in making treatment decisions. By learning from patient data and clinical guidelines, RL models can provide personalized recommendations for diagnosis, treatment plans, and care management. These systems can aid healthcare professionals in decision-making processes, ensuring more informed and evidence-based treatment strategies for Alzheimer's patients.

While RL shows promise in these areas, its application in Alzheimer's research and treatment is still evolving. Further research, validation, and collaboration between AI researchers and healthcare professionals are crucial to ensure the responsible and effective use of RL models in finding and treating Alzheimer's disease [16].

Table 2 presents a comparison of various AI-based Alzheimer's models, including machine learning algorithms, deep learning algorithms, natural language processing models, generative adversarial networks (GANs), and reinforcement learning models. Machine learning algorithms, such as Support Vector Machines (SVM) and Random Forests, offer interpretability and can handle small to medium-sized datasets effectively. Deep learning algorithms, such as Convolutional Neural Networks (CNNs) and Transformers, excel at capturing complex patterns in large datasets but require significant computational resources and labeled data. Natural language processing models, like Word Embeddings and Recurrent Neural Networks (RNNs), are suitable for processing and understanding textual data but may struggle with contextual understanding. Generative Adversarial Networks (GANs) can generate realistic data samples, aiding data augmentation, although training stability can be an issue. Reinforcement learning models, including Deep Q-Networks (DQNs) and Proximal Policy Optimization (PPO), can learn optimal actions based on rewards but demand extensive training and exploration. Determining the best model depends on the specific requirements, available resources, and nature of the problem [17]. There is no universally superior model, as each has its strengths and limitations, and the most suitable choice varies based on the circumstances.

The most effective model among various AI-based Alzheimer's models will vary depending on the particular needs and limitations of the issue at hand. Each model has unique benefits and drawbacks. When choosing the best model for a particular scenario, it is critical to take into account variables including the type of data, the resources at hand, computing needs, and performance goals. The decision should be based on careful examination of the aforementioned aspects because there is no single "best" model that can be used in all situations.

Some of the datasets that are frequently used to train and assess AI-based Alzheimer's models are listed below:

- **Alzheimer's Disease Neuroimaging Initiative (ADNI)**: This dataset contains medical information from over 1,000 persons with Alzheimer's disease and healthy controls, including MRI, PET, and clinical data.

Table 2 A table that summarizes the different types of AI-based Alzheimer's models in more detail and comparison between them:

Model type	Description	Advantages	Disadvantages	Example
Machine Learning Algorithm	A type of algorithm that learns from data and makes predictions	Can be used with a variety of data types	Can be computationally expensive to train	Support vector machines, decision trees, and k-nearest neighbors
Deep Learning Algorithm	A type of machine learning algorithm that uses artificial neural networks to learn from data	Can achieve high accuracy on complex tasks	Can be computationally expensive to train	Convolutional neural networks, recurrent neural networks, deep reinforcement learning
Natural Language Processing Model	A type of machine learning algorithm that can understand and process human language	Can be used to analyze speech recordings and medical records	Can be difficult to train on large datasets	Named entity recognition, sentiment analysis, and machine translation
Generative Adversarial Networks Model	A type of deep learning algorithm that can generate new data that is similar to the data it was trained on	Can be used to generate images of brain tissue that are similar to those of people with Alzheimer's disease	Can be computationally expensive to train	Generating images of brain tissue, generating text that is similar to the writing of people with Alzheimer's disease
Reinforcement Learning Model	A type of machine learning algorithm that learns from trial and error	Can be used to train agents to make decisions in complex environments	Can be difficult to train in some cases	Training agents to make decisions in complex environments

- **The Parkinson's Progression Markers Initiative (PPMI)** collection contains MRI, PET, and clinical information from more than 2,000 people with Parkinson's disease and matched healthy individuals.
- **The ALS-TDI (ALS Therapeutic Development Institute)** dataset contains medical information from more than 10,000 ALS patients.
- **Frontotemporal Dementia-UPF (FTD-UPF)**: This dataset contains clinical information from more than 1,000 FTD sufferers.

16 Conclusion

The advancement of AI has revolutionized the investigation of neurodegenerative diseases like Alzheimer's, Parkinson's, and ALS. By integrating various datasets, such as clinical records, genetic data, neuroimaging scans, and molecular profiles, AI approaches have significantly improved the precision and effectiveness of illness detection. This has led to early detection of illness prodromal symptoms or subtle disease indicators, resulting in more accurate diagnoses. AI-driven diagnostic models have also improved patient outcomes by enabling physicians to make informed decisions based on various data sources. AI-based predictive modeling offers valuable insights into disease course and prognosis, enabling better treatment planning and resource allocation. These models help healthcare providers customize medicines and interventions to meet specific patient requirements. Neuroimaging analysis has shown promise in the detection and management of neurodegenerative disorders, as AI systems can analyze complex data to identify patterns associated with certain diseases or anatomical alterations in the brain. This helps in proper diagnosis and monitoring of the disease's course over time. AI systems can speed up the process of locating viable medication candidates and create more effective clinical trials. AI is capable of predicting drug-target interactions and locating potential therapeutic compounds by quickly evaluating biological databases. This has important implications for the creation of efficient neurodegenerative disease therapies, advancing the search for a cure and improving patient outcomes. AI has the potential to revolutionize the diagnosis, treatment, and management of Alzheimer's disease, as it can uncover hidden patterns and connections within complicated data. Early diagnosis and treatment of the disease can lead to more successful therapies and improved patient outcomes. AI systems can also enhance drug discovery through predictive modeling and virtual screening, allowing for the identification of potential therapeutic compounds and enhancing the drug discovery process.

17 Future Scope

The use of AI in the future for the study of neurodegenerative diseases, notably Alzheimer‘s disease, is extremely promising and offers great promise for improvements in management, therapy, and diagnostics. For a thorough knowledge of neurodegenerative illnesses, the integration of several datasets, including genetic data, neuroimaging scans, clinical records, and wearable device data, offers enormous promise. This multi-modal data may be successfully integrated and analyzed using AI algorithms, revealing intricate linkages and patterns that can help with better diagnosis and treatment planning. AI algorithms may provide precise illness trajectories by examining longitudinal patient data, such as clinical records, neuroimaging scans, and biomarker assessments, enabling improved treatment planning and resource allocation. Explainable AI is becoming important, especially in healthcare applications, as AI algorithms get more and more complicated. AI-powered decision support systems can help medical personnel make well-informed choices by taking a variety of patient-specific characteristics and treatment alternatives into account. The effectiveness and broad application of AI in neurodegenerative illnesses depend critically on cooperation between researchers, healthcare organizations, and technology businesses. The production of large-scale datasets that include a variety of populations and disease subtypes can be facilitated by encouraging data-sharing programs and developing platforms for collaborative study. The use of AI in healthcare presents ethical questions including algorithm bias, data privacy, and patient confidentiality. To retain patient privacy and trust while utilizing the benefits of AI in neurodegenerative illnesses, openness, informed permission, and ethical data governance are crucial. Healthcare personnel may get familiar with AI algorithms and their applications through ongoing education and training programs, facilitating their acceptance and integration into healthcare systems. Using AI to research neurodegenerative diseases, especially Alzheimer's disease, has a wide range of possible applications and has the potential to significantly enhance diagnoses, therapy, and management. Future research should concentrate on developing prediction models for illness progression, explainable AI systems, and the integration of AI algorithms with multi-modal data. We can enhance patient outcomes, customize therapies, and ultimately create a society with a considerably lower incidence of neurodegenerative illnesses by utilizing the potential of AI.

References

1. Shaheen, M. Y. (2021). Applications of Artificial Intelligence (AI) in healthcare: A review. *ScienceOpen Preprints*.
2. Tăuţan, A. M., Ionescu, B., & Santarnecchi, E. (2021). Artificial intelligence in neurodegenerative diseases: A review of available tools with a focus on machine learning techniques. *Artificial Intelligence in Medicine, 117*, 102081.
3. Termine, A., Fabrizio, C., Strafella, C., Caputo, V., Petrosini, L., Caltagirone, C., & Cascella, R. (2021). Multi-layer picture of neurodegenerative diseases: Lessons from the use of big data through artificial intelligence. *Journal of Personalized Medicine, 11*(4), 280.
4. Mathur, S., & Arora, A. (2020). Internet of Things (IoT) and PKI-based security architecture.
5. Khatami, S. G., Mubeen, S., & Hofmann-Apitius, M. (2020). Data science in neurodegenerative disease: Its capabilities, limitations, and perspectives. *Current Opinion in Neurology, 33*(2), 249.
6. Fabrizio, C., Termine, A., Caltagirone, C., & Sancesario, G. (2021). Artificial intelligence for Alzheimer's disease: Promise or challenge? *Diagnostics, 11*(8), 1473.
7. Battista, P., Salvatore, C., Berlingeri, M., Cerasa, A., & Castiglioni, I. (2020). Artificial intelligence and neuropsychological measures: The case of Alzheimer's disease. *Neuroscience & Biobehavioral Reviews, 114*, 211–228.
8. Subasi, A. (2020). Use of artificial intelligence in Alzheimer's disease detection. *Artificial Intelligence in Precision Health*, 257–278.
9. Zhao, X., Ang, C. K. E., Acharya, U. R., & Cheong, K. H. (2021). Application of Artificial Intelligence techniques for the detection of Alzheimer's disease using structural MRI images. *Biocybernetics and Biomedical Engineering, 41*(2), 456–473.

10. Noor, M. B. T., Zenia, N. Z., Kaiser, M. S., Mahmud, M., & Al Mamun, S. (2019). Detecting neurodegenerative disease from MRI: a brief review on a deep learning perspective. In *Brain informatics: 12th international conference, BI 2019, Haikou, China, December 13–15, 2019, Proceedings 12* (pp. 115–125). Springer International Publishing.
11. Mathur, S., Shantanu, A., & Rana, A. (2021). Estimating the imaging in medical science using image processing techniques. *In Journal of Physics: Conference Series* (Vol. 1714, No. 1). IOP Publishing.
12. Mikhalskii, A. I., & Novoseltseva, J. A. (2018). Application of data analysis methods in research of neurodegenerative diseases. In *2018 Eleventh international conference management of large-scale system development (MLSD* (pp. 1–4). IEEE.
13. Shusharina, N., Yukhnenko, D., Botman, S., Sapunov, V., Savinov, V., Kamyshov, G., & Voznyuk, I. (2023). Modern methods of diagnostics and treatment of neurodegenerative diseases and depression. *Diagnostics, 13*(3), 573.
14. Migliore, L. U., Fontana, I., Colognato, R., Coppede, F. A., Siciliano, G. A., & Murri, L. U. (2005). Searching for the role and the most suitable biomarkers of oxidative stress in Alzheimer's disease and other neurodegenerative diseases. *Neurobiology of Aging, 26*(5), 587–595.
15. Mathur, S., Singla, T., Bharat, K., & Rana, A. (2022). AIIOT: Emerging IoT with AI technologies. *A Fusion of Artificial Intelligence and Internet of Things for Emerging Cyber Systems*, 269–291.
16. Mathur, S., & Datta, K. (2021). Prediction of Covid-19 cases in India through machine learning using Python. In *2021 9th international conference on reliability, Infocom technologies and optimization (trends and future directions)(ICRITO)* (pp. 1–6). IEEE.
17. Mathur, S. (2021). Evolving IoT and green IoT in healthcare perspective. *Evolving Role of AI and IoMT in the Healthcare Market*, 175–197.

Role of Artificial Intelligence and Internet of Things in Neurodegenerative Diseases

Sandeep Mathur, Subhangee Bhattacharjee, Sheetal Sehgal, and Richa Shekhar

Abstract Neurodegenerative disorders like ALS, Parkinson's, and Alzheimer's pose challenges to healthcare systems. Their intricate nature results from genetics, environment, and lifestyle. Despite increased understanding, effective treatments remain elusive. Recent advancements in artificial intelligence (AI) and the internet of things (IoT) offer new avenues for diagnosis and therapy. This chapter explores AI and IoT applications in neurodegenerative disorders, focusing on diagnosis. AI can analyze extensive datasets encompassing neuroimaging, genetics, and clinical information, enabling more accurate and rapid diagnoses through machine and deep learning. These tools also facilitate early detection and intervention, transforming healthcare and advancing precision medicine. Addressing technical, ethical, and regulatory issues is essential for responsible AI and IoT integration into neurodegenerative disease research and practice. Overall, AI and IoT have significant potential to revolutionize detection, monitoring, and treatment in this field.

Keywords Neurodegenerative diseases · AI · IoT · Neuroimaging · Prognosis

1 Introduction

Alzheimer's disease, Parkinson's disease, and amyotrophic lateral sclerosis (ALS) are only a few examples of the neurodegenerative disorders that have a substantial impact on world health. These chronic conditions are defined by a steady decline in neuronal structure and function, which results in severe cognitive, motor, and sensory

S. Mathur (✉) · S. Bhattacharjee
Noida International University, Greater Noida, Uttar Pradesh, India
e-mail: sandeep2809@gmail.com

S. Sehgal
BIT Mesra, Off campus, Noida, India
e-mail: sheetal@bitmesra.ac.in

R. Shekhar
Amity University, Noida, India
e-mail: rshekhar@amity.edu

© The Author(s), under exclusive license to Springer Nature Switzerland AG 2024

L. Gaur et al. (eds.), *AI and Neuro-Degenerative Diseases*, Studies in Computational Intelligence 1131, https://doi.org/10.1007/978-3-031-53148-4_2

deficits. The prevalence of neurodegenerative illnesses is predicted to climb sharply as the world's aging population grows, putting enormous demand on healthcare systems and calling for novel ways to diagnosis, treatment, and management. The fusion of artificial intelligence and the internet of things has recently become a transformational force in the healthcare industry. AI, which includes machine learning, deep learning, and natural language processing, allows computers to simulate human intelligence and make predictions and judgments based on data [1]. On the other hand, the IoT includes attaching commonplace gadgets and items to the internet to enable smooth data transfer and communication. The combination of AI and IoT could transform how diseases are understood, detected, monitored, and treated when used in the context of neurodegenerative disorders. Numerous prospects exist in the field of neurodegenerative illnesses as a result of the integration of AI and IoT technology [2]. To find illness biomarkers, forecast disease progression, and aid in early diagnosis, AI systems can scan enormous volumes of patient data, including clinical records, genomic data, medical pictures, and data from wearable sensors. This skill has the potential to significantly improve patient outcomes by allowing clinicians to intervene early in the course of the disease. Furthermore, IoT devices, such as wearable sensors, smart home systems, and mobile applications, can collect continuous, real-time data on patients' vital signs, motor function, sleep patterns, and cognitive performance. These devices facilitate remote monitoring and enable healthcare professionals to closely track disease progression and treatment responses [3]. When combined with AI analytics, this data can offer insightful information about illness trends, the efficacy of treatments, and individualized patient care. However, there are obstacles to overcome in order to successfully integrate AI and IoT in the context of neurodegenerative illnesses. To ensure the responsible and ethical use of patient data, ethical issues like as patient privacy, data security, and permission must be carefully considered. Additionally, for seamless integration and collaboration between healthcare practitioners, researchers, and AI systems, the interoperability and standardization of devices, platforms, and data formats are essential. The goal of this research article is to present a thorough analysis of the most recent developments, uses, and difficulties associated with applying AI and IoT technologies in the context of neurodegenerative illnesses. By exploring the potential of AI algorithms for accurate diagnosis, disease prediction, and drug discovery, as well as the integration of IoT devices for remote monitoring and real-time data collection, This study aims to shed light on how these technologies can improve people's lives and make them better for those who suffer from neurodegenerative disorders. In summary, the fusion of AI and IoT has enormous potential to transform the study of neurodegenerative disorders. Healthcare practitioners can obtain deeper insights into illness progression, facilitate early identification, tailor treatment approaches, and enable remote monitoring by leveraging the capabilities of AI algorithms and IoT devices. To guarantee the responsible and successful application of these technologies, it is essential to resolve ethical, statutory, and technical issues. By publishing this study, we hope to advance further investigation into the use of AI and IoT in neurodegenerative illnesses and add to the body of knowledge in this area.

2 Literature Review

Table 1 focuses on the advancements in the diagnosis and treatment of neurodegenerative diseases using AI.

3 Rate of Cases of Neurodegenerative Diseases

Given their rising frequency and incidence, neurodegenerative disorders represent a substantial global health challenge. In recent years, there has been growing concern about the prevalence of neurodegenerative disorders such as ALS, Parkinson's disease, Alzheimer's disease, and Huntington's disease. Millions of people throughout the world are afflicted by Alzheimer's disease, the most prevalent neurological illness. Global estimates predict a significant increase in the number of people with Alzheimer's disease during the next few decades. The prevalence of this disorder is increasing as a result of factors including an aging population, longer life expectancies, and changing lifestyles. According to the World Health Organization (WHO), there are roughly 50 million cases of dementia globally, with 60–70% of those cases being caused by Alzheimer's disease. Parkinson's disease, another prevalent neurodegenerative disorder, also exhibits an increasing trend in the number of cases. It is estimated that more than 6 million individuals globally are living with Parkinson's disease, and this number is expected to double by 2040. The aging population, environmental factors, and genetic predisposition contribute to the rising incidence and prevalence of Parkinson's disease similarly, the rate of cases for other neurodegenerative diseases, such as Huntington's disease and ALS, although relatively lower compared to Alzheimer's and Parkinson's, remains a concern. Huntington's disease is a hereditary disorder, and while it is less common than other neurodegenerative diseases, its impact on affected individuals and their families is substantial. The prevalence of ALS is estimated to be around 2–3 cases per 100,000 individuals worldwide, with varying rates across different regions. It is important to note that accurately determining the rate of neurodegenerative diseases is challenging due to factors such as underreporting, misdiagnosis, and regional variations in healthcare access and diagnostic capabilities. However, studies and population-based surveys provide valuable insights into the increasing burden of these diseases on societies worldwide. The rising rate of cases of neurodegenerative diseases poses significant challenges to healthcare systems, caregivers, and affected individuals. It underscores the urgent need for increased research, early detection strategies, improved access to specialized care, and the development of effective interventions to mitigate the impact of these debilitating conditions. Collaboration between researchers, healthcare professionals, policymakers, and advocacy organizations is crucial to address the growing burden of neurodegenerative diseases and improve the quality of life for individuals affected by these conditions (Fig. 1).

Table 1 Reviewing multiple authors' previous research work

Serial no	Experiment	Author	Outcome	Future directions	References
1	"AI Engineering: Realizing the Potential of AI"	"Jan Bosch, Helena Holmström Olsson, Bjorn Brinne, & Ivica Crnkovic."	AI engineering plays a crucial role in realizing the potential of AI by bridging the gap between AI research and its practical applications	The future directions of AI engineering include the development of explainable AI models	[1]
2	"Neurodegenerative diseases and their related treatment"	Jim Ziyan Xin	It examines various treatment options including medications, therapies, surgical interventions, gene therapy, stem cell therapy	Precision medicine approaches based on individual characteristics, identification of novel therapeutic targets	[2]
3	"AI vs. "AI": Synthetic Minds or Speech Acts"	"Peter R. Lewis, Stephen Marsh, & Jeremy Pitt"	Exploration of the distinction between AI systems that possess true synthetic minds versus those that merely simulate human-like speech acts	It delves into the philosophical and conceptual implications of understanding AI intelligence	[3]
4	"AI-Driven Performance Modelling for AI Inference Workloads"	"Max Sponner, Bernd Waschneck, & Akash Kumar"	Focus is on utilizing AI techniques to develop performance models for AI inference workloads	Future directions include refining performance models, exploring optimization techniques	[4]
5	"IoT and PKI based Security Architecture"	"Sandeep Mathur, Ankita Arora.="	IoT yields significant outcomes across various domains, including enhanced operational efficiency	The future of the IoT will involve its continued expansion across industries	[5]

(continued)

Table 1 (continued)

Serial no	Experiment	Author	Outcome	Future directions	References
6	"The Diversity of AI"	"David B. Leake"	Examination of various dimensions of diversity in AI	The paper emphasizes the significance of diverse datasets, algorithms, and perspectives in AI development	[6]
7	"Sleep and neurodegenerative diseases"	"Masud Husain"	It explores the impact of disrupted sleep on the development and progression of conditions	Investigating the mechanisms linking sleep and neurodegenerative diseases	[7]
8	"Immunotherapies for Neurodegenerative Diseases"	"Ibrahim Mortada, Raymond Farah, & et al."	The paper investigates the role of the immune system in neurodegeneration	The paper emphasizes the need for future research and development in several key areas	[8]
9	"Proteotoxicity and Neurodegenerative Diseases"	"Clara Ruz, Jose Luis Alcantud, & et al."	The paper investigates how protein misfolding, aggregation, and accumulation	The paper emphasizes the need for future investigations and interventions in various areas	[9]
10	"Accelerating AI"	"Vasileios Don Monroe"	Focus is on techniques and methodologies aimed at accelerating AI algorithms and models	Aim is to advance AI acceleration by developing specialized hardware, optimizing algorithms	[10]

4 Impact of AI on Neurodegenerative Diseases

The impact of AI on neurodegenerative diseases has been transformative, revolutionizing in both research and clinical practice. AI technologies have significantly enhanced our understanding of these complex conditions by analyzing vast amounts of data and uncovering patterns and correlations that were previously difficult to identify. Machine learning algorithms trained on diverse datasets, including medical images, genetic information, and clinical records, have demonstrated remarkable accuracy in the early detection and precise diagnosis of neurodegenerative diseases [4]. This early detection enables healthcare professionals to intervene at an earlier

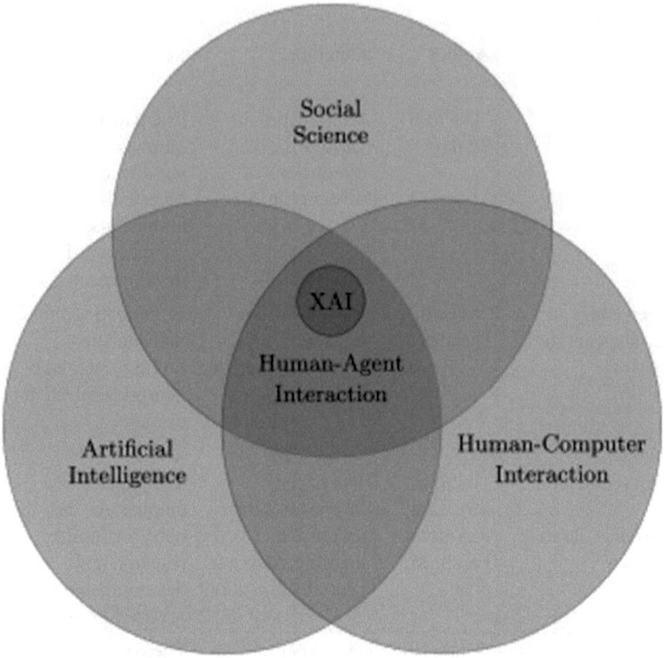

Fig. 1 Scope of explainable AI. "Explanation in AI: Insights from the social sciences", Tim Miller (2019)

stage, providing patients with the opportunity for timely treatment and interventions that may slow disease progression and improve outcomes. Furthermore, AI has facilitated the development of personalized treatment plans tailored to each patient's unique characteristics, disease stage, and response to therapy. By analyzing extensive patient data, including clinical parameters, genetic profiles, and treatment outcomes, AI algorithms can identify optimal treatment strategies and predict the efficacy of different interventions. This individualized approach improves treatment precision and enhances patient outcomes, optimizing their care and quality of life. In addition to diagnosis and treatment, AI has played a significant role in providing ongoing support and care to individuals with neurodegenerative diseases. Virtual assistants and chat bots powered by AI algorithms can offer continuous support, delivering personalized information, medication reminders, and emotional assistance. These systems can engage patients in cognitive training exercises, helping to mitigate cognitive decline and maintain mental acuity. AI-driven robotics and smart devices have also been developed to assist patients with daily activities, enhancing their independence and overall well-being. However, as with any emerging technology, the integration of AI in neurodegenerative diseases is not without challenges. Ethical considerations, such as data privacy and security, informed consent, and algorithmic bias, must be carefully addressed. Furthermore, the successful implementation of

AI in clinical settings requires collaboration among researchers, healthcare professionals, policymakers, and technology developers. In conclusion, the impact of AI on neurodegenerative diseases has been transformative, offering new avenues for early detection, precise diagnosis, personalized treatment, and ongoing support. By harnessing the power of AI, we have the potential to improve patient outcomes, advance scientific understanding, and ultimately find effective treatments and interventions for neurodegenerative diseases. However, it is essential to navigate the ethical and implementation challenges associated with AI to ensure responsible and equitable integration into healthcare systems and maximize its benefits for patients worldwide.

5 Impact of IoT on Neurodegenerative Diseases

The impact of the IoT on neurodegenerative diseases has brought about a paradigm shift in healthcare, offering unprecedented opportunities for personalized and proactive management of these complex conditions. IoT devices have revolutionized data collection by enabling continuous monitoring of various health parameters. Wearable sensors, for instance, track vital signs, movement patterns, and sleep quality, providing a comprehensive view of patients' well-being. This continuous stream of data, combined with the power of advanced analytics, opens up new avenues for early detection, precise diagnosis, and tailored interventions. Healthcare professionals can now leverage IoT-generated data to identify subtle changes in disease progression, detect early warning signs of complications, and intervene promptly to optimize treatment outcomes. Additionally, IoT facilitates remote monitoring and telemedicine, allowing individuals with neurodegenerative diseases to receive specialized care and support from the comfort of their own homes. Through virtual consultations and telehealth platforms, healthcare providers can remotely assess patients' condition, offer timely guidance, and adjust treatment plans as needed. This not only improves access to specialized care but also enhances patient convenience, reduces the burden of frequent hospital visits, and promotes active engagement in self-management. Furthermore, IoT empowers patients by providing them with real-time insights into their health, fostering self-awareness, and enabling them to actively participate in their own care. The integration of IoT in neurodegenerative disease management has the potential to revolutionize the healthcare landscape, improving patient outcomes, enhancing quality of life, and paving the way for personalized and patient-centric approaches to care.

6 Integration of IoT with AI in the Context of Neurodegenerative Diseases

The integration of the IoT with AI holds immense promise for transforming the management of neurodegenerative diseases. IoT devices, such as wearable sensors, smart home technology, and remote monitoring systems, provide a wealth of real-time data that can be harnessed to improve patient care [5]. These devices capture diverse information such as vital signs, physical activity, sleep patterns, medication adherence, and environmental factors, creating a comprehensive picture of a patient's health status. By integrating this IoT-generated data with AI algorithms, healthcare professionals can unlock powerful insights and derive meaningful patterns that may otherwise go unnoticed. The integration of IoT with AI presents numerous opportunities for enhancing the management of neurodegenerative diseases:

6.1 *Remote Monitoring and Telemedicine*

The integration of IoT with AI has revolutionized remote monitoring and telemedicine for individuals with neurodegenerative diseases. Through IoT devices, such as wearable sensors and smart home technology, real-time data on vital signs, movement patterns, medication adherence, and environmental factors can be continuously collected and transmitted. AI algorithms then analyze this data, providing valuable insights to healthcare professionals for remote monitoring and proactive decision-making [6]. This capability has significant implications for individuals with neurodegenerative diseases who may face challenges in accessing specialized care or have difficulty with frequent hospital visits. Remote monitoring and telemedicine enable healthcare providers to remotely assess patients' health status, track disease progression, and intervene in a timely manner. They can review the IoT-generated data, identify deviations from normal patterns, and provide appropriate guidance or interventions, ensuring optimal disease management and reducing the risk of complications. Furthermore, telemedicine allows for virtual consultations and remote follow-ups, enabling individuals to receive specialized care from the comfort of their homes. This integration enhances patient convenience, improves access to healthcare, and empowers individuals with neurodegenerative diseases to actively participate in their own care, leading to better outcomes and improved quality of life.

6.2 *Predictive Analytics and Early Intervention*

The integration of IoT with AI enables powerful predictive analytics and early intervention strategies in the management of neurodegenerative diseases. By leveraging the continuous data collected through IoT devices, such as wearable sensors and smart home technology, AI algorithms can analyze patterns, detect subtle changes, and predict disease progression or the onset of complications. This predictive capability empowers healthcare professionals to intervene at an early stage, allowing for proactive measures and personalized treatment plans. For example, AI algorithms can analyze movement patterns and activity data collected through IoT devices to detect changes in gait, mobility, or coordination that may indicate a decline in motor function. By identifying these changes early on, healthcare professionals can intervene with targeted therapies, exercise regimens, or assistive devices to mitigate functional decline and enhance patient outcomes. Predictive analytics also allow for personalized interventions based on individual characteristics and response to treatment, improving the efficacy and efficiency of care provided. By embracing early intervention strategies driven by predictive analytics, the integration of IoT with AI holds the potential to significantly impact the course of neurodegenerative diseases, enabling timely interventions and ultimately improving the quality of life for individuals affected by these conditions.

6.3 Personalized Rehabilitation and Therapy

The integration of IoT with AI has opened up new possibilities for personalized rehabilitation and therapy for individuals with neurodegenerative diseases. IoT devices, such as smart wearable and assistive technologies, capture real-time movement and activity data, which can be analyzed by AI algorithms to provide tailored rehabilitation and therapy programs. By continuously monitoring and analyzing the data, AI algorithms can track progress, identify areas for improvement, and customize treatment plans based on individual needs and abilities. For instance, AI algorithms can analyze sensor data to assess motor function, range of motion, and muscle strength, enabling personalized exercise regimens and adaptive therapy interventions. Furthermore, AI can adapt therapy programs in real-time, making necessary adjustments based on individual progress or changes in disease status. This personalized approach to rehabilitation and therapy optimizes outcomes by tailoring interventions to the specific needs and capabilities of each individual, improving functional abilities, promoting independence, and enhancing the overall quality of life for individuals with neurodegenerative diseases.

6.4 Data-Driven Research and Drug Development

The integration of IoT with AI offers unprecedented opportunities for data-driven research and drug development in the field of neurodegenerative diseases. IoT devices capture a vast amount of real-time data, including patient characteristics, lifestyle factors, symptom profiles, and treatment responses. AI algorithms can analyze and interpret this data to uncover novel insights, identify patterns, and accelerate research efforts. By aggregating and analyzing data from a large number of individuals, AI algorithms can help researchers better understand disease mechanisms, identify subtypes within neurodegenerative diseases, and discover new biomarkers that could facilitate early diagnosis and targeted interventions. Furthermore, AI algorithms can assist in the identification of potential drug targets and the development of novel therapeutic approaches. By analyzing large datasets and combining various sources of information, including genomic data, clinical records, and treatment outcomes, AI can contribute to the discovery and development of innovative treatments and personalized medicine approaches. This data-driven research facilitated by the integration of IoT with AI has the potential to revolutionize our understanding of neurodegenerative diseases and expedite the development of effective therapies, ultimately improving the lives of individuals affected by these conditions.

6.5 Caregiver Support and Assistance

The integration of IoT with AI brings forth significant benefits in terms of caregiver support and assistance for individuals with neurodegenerative diseases. Caregivers play a vital role in providing care and support to individuals affected by these conditions, often facing numerous challenges and responsibilities. IoT devices integrated with AI algorithms can provide invaluable assistance to caregivers, offering guidance, resources, and real-time updates on their loved ones' health status. Caregivers can leverage IoT-enabled devices and AI-powered virtual assistants to receive personalized care giving techniques, educational materials, and alerts for emergencies or changes in the patient's condition[7]. These intelligent systems can offer support for medication management, reminders for appointments or activities, and advice on managing behavioural and psychological symptoms. The integration of IoT with AI thus alleviates caregiver burden, enhances their ability to provide optimal care, and improves their overall well-being. By leveraging these technologies, caregivers can feel more supported and equipped to provide effective care, leading to improved outcomes for both the caregiver and the individual with neurodegenerative diseases.

6.6 Population Health Management

The integration of IoT with AI has significant implications for population health management in the field of neurodegenerative diseases. By leveraging the vast amount of data collected through IoT devices, AI algorithms can provide valuable insights into disease trends, risk factors, and population-level health indicators. This data-driven approach enables healthcare systems to track the prevalence and incidence of neurodegenerative diseases, identify high-risk populations, and design targeted interventions and preventive strategies. AI algorithms can analyze aggregated data from IoT devices to detect patterns and correlations, facilitating early identification of individuals at risk of developing neurodegenerative diseases. This population-level analysis supports public health efforts by enabling the implementation of proactive measures, such as health education campaigns, lifestyle interventions, and screening programs. Moreover, AI algorithms can continuously analyze population-level data to evaluate the effectiveness of interventions, monitor outcomes, and refine population health management strategies. The integration of IoT with AI in population health management enhances our ability to understand and address the complex challenges posed by neurodegenerative diseases, ultimately leading to improved health outcomes and better quality of life for the affected populations.

AI algorithms, trained on large datasets and capable of complex pattern recognition, can analyze the IoT data to detect subtle changes in disease progression, predict exacerbations, and identify potential interventions. For example, by monitoring gait patterns and movement data through IoT devices, AI algorithms can identify deviations and detect early signs of mobility decline in neurodegenerative diseases such as Parkinson's or multiple sclerosis. This enables timely interventions, such as adjustments in medication or referral to physical therapy, to mitigate functional decline and enhance patient outcomes. Moreover, the integration of IoT and AI enables personalized treatment planning for individuals with neurodegenerative diseases. By continuously monitoring patient data through IoT devices, AI algorithms can analyze the effectiveness of different interventions, adjust treatment plans in real-time, and provide personalized recommendations [8]. For instance, AI can identify optimal medication dosages based on patient response, recognize potential adverse reactions, and suggest alternative approaches, all while considering individual patient characteristics and disease progression. In addition to monitoring and treatment, IoT and AI can facilitate remote patient support and caregiver assistance. IoT devices can transmit data to AI-powered virtual assistants or chatbots, providing round-the-clock monitoring, education, and emotional support. These virtual assistants can deliver personalized information, reminders, and guidance to patients, empowering them to actively engage in their self-care. Caregivers can also benefit from IoT and AI integration by receiving real-time updates on their loved ones' health status, ensuring timely interventions and reducing caregiver burden.

However, the integration of IoT with AI in the context of neurodegenerative diseases does come with challenges. Privacy and security of patient data are paramount, necessitating robust safeguards and adherence to regulatory guidelines. Interoperability among different IoT devices and standardization of data formats are crucial to ensure seamless integration and effective data sharing. Ethical considerations, including informed consent, data ownership, and transparency in AI decision-making, must also be addressed to maintain patient trust and ensure responsible implementation. In conclusion, the integration of IoT with AI in the management of neurodegenerative diseases has tremendous potential to revolutionize patient care. By leveraging the real-time data captured by IoT devices and applying AI algorithms, healthcare professionals can gain valuable insights, personalize treatment plans, and provide continuous support to patients. While challenges remain, addressing these issues through collaborative efforts will enable the realization of the full benefits of IoT and AI integration in improving the lives of individuals living with neurodegenerative diseases.

7 AI Algorithms on Neurodegenerative Diseases

AI algorithms have emerged as transformative tools in the field of neurodegenerative diseases, offering unprecedented opportunities for diagnosis, prognosis, and personalized treatment. With the ability to analyze vast amounts of data, including medical imaging, genomics, clinical records, and wearable sensor data, AI algorithms can extract valuable insights and patterns that may not be readily apparent to human observers. These algorithms utilize advanced machine learning techniques, such as deep learning and reinforcement learning, to uncover hidden relationships and detect subtle changes in disease progression. In terms of diagnosis, AI algorithms have shown great promise in aiding early detection by identifying specific biomarkers and patterns that may indicate the presence of neurodegenerative diseases. Through the analysis of medical imaging data, such as magnetic resonance imaging (MRI) scans and positron emission tomography (PET) scans, AI algorithms can identify characteristic brain changes associated with conditions like Alzheimer's disease, Parkinson's disease, and multiple sclerosis. This early detection allows for timely interventions and the initiation of appropriate treatment strategies, potentially leading to better patient outcomes. Furthermore, AI algorithms contribute to the prognostication of neurodegenerative diseases by predicting disease progression and estimating future functional decline. By analyzing longitudinal data from diverse sources, such as clinical assessments, imaging studies, and patient-reported outcomes, AI algorithms can generate personalized prognostic models that take into account individual characteristics, genetic profiles, and environmental factors. These models help healthcare professionals anticipate disease trajectory, inform care planning, and facilitate discussions around prognosis with patients and their families. Personalized treatment approaches are another area where AI algorithms demonstrate their potential. By integrating various data sources, including genomic profiles, clinical data, medication responses, and lifestyle factors, AI algorithms can create patient-specific models to guide treatment decisions. For instance, AI algorithms can analyze genetic data to predict drug responses and identify potential adverse reactions, enabling personalized medication regimens for individuals with neurodegenerative diseases [10]. AI algorithms can also assist in optimizing therapeutic interventions by analyzing data from wearable sensors and remote monitoring devices, which capture real-time data on vital signs, movement patterns, and sleep quality. This continuous monitoring allows for personalized adjustments to treatment plans based on the patient's dynamic health status. In addition to diagnosis and treatment, AI algorithms contribute to the development of innovative therapies for neurodegenerative diseases. By leveraging large-scale datasets, AI algorithms can identify novel drug targets, design targeted therapies, and facilitate the discovery of potential disease-modifying treatments.

Through the integration of genomic data, protein interaction networks, and computational modelling, AI algorithms enable researchers to accelerate the identification and validation of promising therapeutic candidates. This can significantly expedite the drug discovery and development process, potentially leading to more effective and tailored treatments for individuals with neurodegenerative diseases. While AI algorithms offer immense potential, challenges remain in their implementation. Ensuring the privacy and security of patient data, addressing biases in algorithms, and establishing regulatory frameworks are critical considerations to mitigate risks and ensure responsible deployment of AI technologies in the field of neurodegenerative diseases. In conclusion, AI algorithms hold tremendous promise in the realm of neurodegenerative diseases. With their ability to analyze complex datasets, detect patterns, and provide personalized insights, these algorithms have the potential to revolutionize diagnosis, prognostication, and treatment approaches. By leveraging AI, healthcare professionals can improve early detection, optimize care plans, and pave the way for innovative therapies, ultimately enhancing the lives of individuals affected by neurodegenerative diseases.

8 Potential of AI in the Field of Neurodegenerative Diseases

The potential of AI in the field of neurodegenerative diseases is vast and holds transformative possibilities across various aspects of disease management. AI algorithms have the capacity to analyze large and diverse datasets, encompassing medical imaging, genomic information, clinical records, and wearable sensor data. By leveraging machine learning techniques, AI algorithms can uncover complex patterns, detect subtle changes, and extract meaningful insights that can significantly impact the diagnosis, treatment, and overall management of neurodegenerative diseases. One key area where AI shows tremendous potential is in early detection and accurate diagnosis. AI algorithms can process and analyze medical imaging data, such as magnetic resonance imaging (MRI) scans, positron emission tomography (PET) scans, and functional MRI (fMRI) data, to detect and interpret subtle changes in brain structure and function. This enables the identification of early biomarkers and the differentiation between various neurodegenerative diseases, aiding in the timely initiation of interventions and personalized treatment plans. Furthermore, AI algorithms can predict disease progression and provide valuable prognostic information. By integrating longitudinal clinical data, imaging findings, and genetic profiles, AI algorithms can develop predictive models that estimate the rate of disease progression and anticipate future functional decline. This information allows healthcare professionals to tailor treatment plans, optimize care strategies, and provide patients and their families with more accurate prognostic information, ultimately enhancing decision-making and patient outcomes [11].

In addition to diagnosis and prognosis, AI holds great promise in the development of innovative therapies for neurodegenerative diseases. By leveraging AI algorithms and computational models, researchers can expedite the process of identifying potential drug targets and designing targeted therapies. AI facilitates the analysis of genomic data, molecular pathways, and protein–protein interactions, enabling the discovery of novel therapeutic candidates and the development of precision medicine approaches. This not only enhances the potential for disease modification but also allows for the customization of treatments based on individual patient characteristics and genetic profiles. AI technologies, such as remote monitoring and telemedicine, have the potential to revolutionize disease management and patient care for individuals with neurodegenerative diseases. IoT devices and wearable sensors equipped with AI algorithms enable continuous monitoring of vital signs, movement patterns, sleep quality, and medication adherence. This real-time data can be remotely accessed by healthcare professionals, facilitating personalized interventions, early detection of complications, and timely adjustments to treatment plans. Telemedicine platforms powered by AI algorithms enable virtual consultations, remote patient monitoring, and the delivery of specialized care to individuals in remote or underserved areas. These technologies enhance access to healthcare, reduce the burden of frequent hospital visits, and empower patients to actively participate in their own care. However, to fully realize the potential of AI in neurodegenerative diseases, certain challenges must be addressed. Ensuring the privacy and security of patient data is paramount, as AI relies on access to sensitive health information. Additionally, addressing algorithmic biases and ensuring the transparency and interpretability of AI algorithms is crucial to building trust and ethical implementation. Regulatory frameworks need to be developed to guide the responsible use of AI technologies in healthcare settings and to ensure adherence to ethical standards. In conclusion, the potential of AI in neurodegenerative diseases is vast and holds promise for revolutionizing disease management. From early detection and accurate diagnosis to the development of innovative therapies and personalized treatment approaches, AI algorithms have the capacity to transform patient care, enhance outcomes, and improve the quality of life for individuals affected by neurodegenerative diseases. It is imperative that ongoing research, collaboration, and ethical considerations continue to shape the implementation of AI in this critical field of healthcare. The following Fig. 2 shows inflammasome activation in neurodegenerative disease.

9 The Role of IoT in Neurodegenerative Diseases

The importance of IoT in the context of neurodegenerative diseases cannot be overstated. It brings innovative solutions to address the unique challenges faced by both individuals and healthcare professionals in handling these complex conditions. IoT plays a versatile role that includes things like remote monitoring, personalized care, continuous tracking, support for caregivers, and data-based research. This transforms how we manage diseases, betters patient care, and propels advancements in the field. One significant role of IoT is making remote monitoring and telemedicine possible, which is a game-changer for people dealing with neurodegenerative diseases. Devices like wearable sensors, smart home tech, and remote monitoring systems let us gather

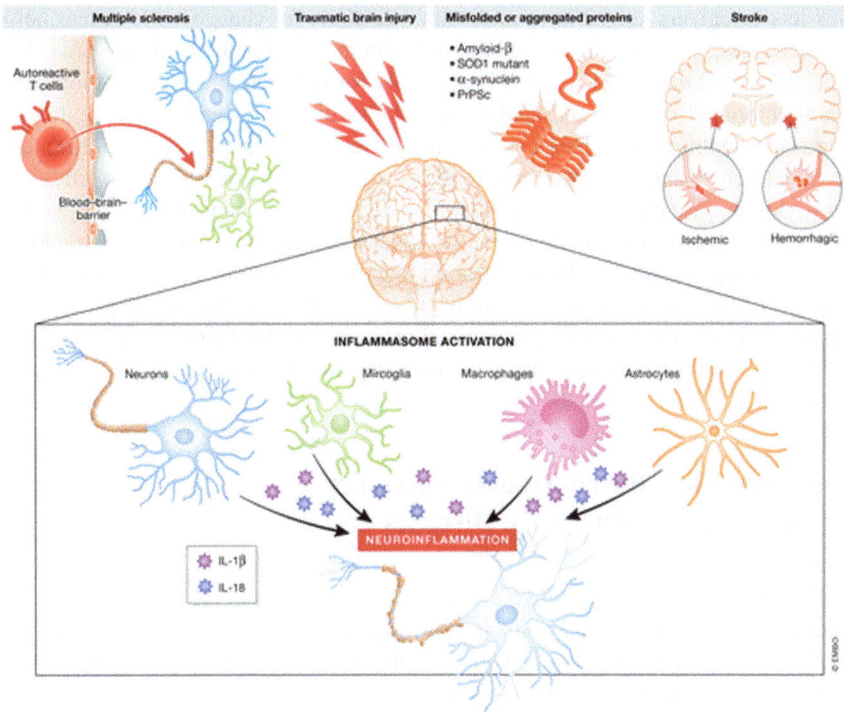

Fig. 2 Inflammasome activation in neurodegenerative disease, "Inflammasomes in neuroinflammatory and neurodegenerative diseases", S. Voet, M. Lamkanfi, (2019)

real-time health data—heart rate, blood pressure, movement, sleep, and medication adherence. Healthcare experts can access this data remotely to keep tabs on patients, spot changes, and provide timely help. This lessens the need for frequent hospital visits, especially important for those in remote areas or with limited mobility. Thanks to IoT-powered telemedicine, virtual check-ups and specialized care can happen, improving accessibility and convenience. Moreover, IoT shines in offering personalized care that suits each individual's needs. By gathering data from IoT devices and using smart analytics and AI, healthcare professionals gain insights into patients' unique profiles, genetics, how they respond to meds, and lifestyle. With all this info, they can create personalized treatment and care plans that give the best results and quality of life. Personalized care empowers patients to take charge of their health and stick to treatments. Continuous monitoring is also vital in neurodegenerative diseases, where symptoms can change often. IoT devices provide real-time data that helps healthcare pros track disease progression, spot patterns, and catch early signs. Devices like wearables and smart home tools track vital signs, movement, and sleep, allowing proactive interventions and prompt adjustments to treatment plans. IoT also does a lot to support caregivers and patients. Caregivers of people with neurodegenerative diseases face many challenges, but IoT offers remote access to patient data.

This lets caregivers keep an eye on health, get alerts for changes, and access help. It eases stress, improves care, and boosts communication with healthcare pros. The data gathered through IoT devices is also gold for research and drug development. When combined with AI and analytics, it shows disease patterns, how treatments work, and health trends. This kind of data-driven research helps find biomarkers, new treatments, and innovative interventions, speeding up scientific discoveries and improving disease management. In closing, IoT is a game-changer in neurodegenerative diseases. It brings remote monitoring, personalized care, continuous tracking, caregiver support, and data-based research together, improving treatment outcomes, quality of life, and our understanding of these complex conditions. Integrating IoT can revolutionize disease management, enhance care, and drive progress in the field, making life better for those affected by neurodegenerative diseases.

10 Ai and IoT Based Models Necessary for Neurodegenerative Diseases

In the realm of neurodegenerative diseases, the integration of AI and IoT models is crucial for advancing disease management, improving patient outcomes, and facilitating research. Various AI and IoT models play a vital role in addressing the unique challenges associated with these conditions:

10.1 Machine Learning and Deep Learning Models

AI algorithms, including machine learning and deep learning models, are essential for analyzing complex datasets in neurodegenerative diseases. These models can identify patterns, detect biomarkers, and predict disease progression based on diverse data sources such as medical imaging, genomics, and clinical records. By leveraging machine learning and deep learning algorithms, accurate diagnosis, prognosis, and personalized treatment planning can be achieved, thereby enhancing patient care.

10.2 Remote Monitoring and Wearable Devices

IoT models, in combination with wearable devices, enable remote monitoring of individuals with neurodegenerative diseases. These devices capture real-time data on vital signs, movement patterns, sleep quality, and medication adherence. IoT models facilitate the integration of this data into comprehensive health records, allowing healthcare professionals to monitor disease progression, detect changes, and intervene proactively. Remote monitoring enhances accessibility to care, reduces the burden of frequent hospital visits, and empowers patients to actively participate in their own health management.

10.3 Telemedicine Platforms

IoT-enabled telemedicine platforms play a critical role in providing remote access to specialized care for individuals with neurodegenerative diseases. These platforms facilitate virtual consultations, remote patient monitoring, and real-time communication between healthcare providers and patients. AI algorithms integrated into telemedicine models aid in accurate interpretation of patient data, assist in diagnosing and managing symptoms, and optimize treatment plans. Telemedicine platforms improve healthcare access, particularly for individuals in remote or underserved areas, and enable timely interventions.

10.4 Data Analytics and Predictive Models

AI and IoT models enable the analysis of large-scale datasets in neurodegenerative diseases, supporting data-driven research and predictive modelling. By integrating various data sources, including clinical records, genetic profiles, and environmental factors, predictive models can estimate disease progression, assess treatment responses, and identify potential risk factors. Data analytics and predictive models provide valuable insights for healthcare professionals, researchers, and policymakers, contributing to evidence-based decision-making and advancements in disease management.

10.5 Smart Home Technology

IoT models integrated with smart home technology offer innovative solutions for neurodegenerative diseases. These models incorporate sensors and devices throughout the home environment to monitor safety, activities of daily living, and environmental factors [12]. AI algorithms analyze the collected data to identify potential hazards, detect abnormal behaviours, and provide personalized recommendations for improving home safety and quality of life. Smart home technology enhances independence, reduces caregiver burden, and supports aging in place for individuals with neurodegenerative diseases.

10.6 Data Security and Privacy Models

Given the sensitive nature of health data, robust data security and privacy models are essential when implementing AI and IoT in neurodegenerative diseases. These models ensure the protection of patient information, secure data transmission, and compliance with privacy regulations. Effective security measures, such as encryption, access controls, and secure data storage, are crucial to maintain patient trust and confidentiality.

In summary, the integration of AI and IoT models is necessary for comprehensive disease management in neurodegenerative diseases. These models encompass machine learning algorithms, remote monitoring, telemedicine platforms, data analytics, smart home technology, and robust data security measures. The integration of AI and IoT in neurodegenerative diseases has the potential to revolutionize patient care, improve outcomes, and advance our understanding of these complex conditions.

11 Technologies Used for Neurodegenerative Diseases

The integration of AI and IoT technologies in neurodegenerative diseases offers innovative solutions for early detection, personalized treatment, continuous monitoring, and improved patient care. The following technologies in Table 2 play a crucial role in enhancing disease management and supporting individuals living with neurodegenerative diseases. These technologies are IoT and AI based which are primary in the field of Neurodegenerative diseases. However there are many more AI and IoT based technologies that are used other than the ones mentioned here.

12 Opportunities Provided by AI and IoT in Neurodegenerative Diseases

The integration of AI and the IoT offers a range of opportunities in the management of neurodegenerative diseases. These technologies have the potential to transform disease diagnosis, treatment, monitoring, and overall patient care. Here are some key opportunities provided by AI and IoT in neurodegenerative diseases:

12.1 Early Detection and Diagnosis

AI algorithms can analyze diverse data sources, including medical imaging, genetic profiles, and clinical records, to identify early biomarkers and patterns associated with

Table 2 Technologies used for neurodegenerative diseases

Technology	Description	Uses
Machine Learning	Utilizes algorithms to learn patterns from data	- Early diagnosis and detection of neurodegenerative diseases - Predicting disease progression - Identifying biomarkers for personalized treatment
Deep Learning	A subset of machine learning utilizing neural networks	- Analysis of complex medical imaging data (MRI, PET scans) to detect disease-related patterns - Automated interpretation of medical images - Predicting disease outcomes
Wearable Devices	IoT devices worn on the body to collect real-time data	- Continuous monitoring of vital signs (heart rate, blood pressure) - Movement tracking for assessing motor symptoms - Sleep quality monitoring
Smart Home Technology	IoT devices integrated into home environment	- Monitoring activities of daily living (ADLs) - Assisting with home safety and fall detection - Providing reminders and prompts for medication adherence
Telemedicine Platforms	IoT-enabled platforms for remote healthcare delivery	- Remote consultations and virtual visits - Monitoring and management of symptoms from a distance - Access to specialized care for patients in remote areas
Data Analytics	Analyzing large-scale datasets for insights	- Identifying disease patterns and risk factors - Predictive modelling for disease progression and treatment response - Population health management
Robotics	AI-powered robots assisting with daily tasks	- Assisting individuals with mobility impairments - Supporting rehabilitation and therapy - Providing companionship and cognitive stimulation

neurodegenerative diseases. By leveraging machine learning and deep learning techniques, AI can assist in the early detection and accurate diagnosis of these conditions, enabling timely interventions and personalized treatment plans.

12.2 Personalized Treatment and Care

AI and IoT technologies enable personalized treatment approaches for individuals with neurodegenerative diseases. By integrating data from wearable devices, sensors, and patient records, AI algorithms can provide insights into individual patient profiles, genetic information, medication responses, and lifestyle factors. This facilitates tailored treatment plans, optimizing interventions to suit specific needs and improving therapeutic outcomes.

12.3 Continuous Monitoring and Remote Care

IoT devices, such as wearable sensors and smart home technology, allow for continuous monitoring of vital signs, movement patterns, and sleep quality. Real-time data collected from these devices can be remotely accessed by healthcare professionals, enabling proactive interventions and remote care delivery. This enhances accessibility to healthcare services, reduces the need for frequent hospital visits, and empowers patients to actively participate in their own care.

12.4 Predictive Analytics and Disease Progression

AI algorithms, when combined with longitudinal clinical data, imaging findings, and genetic profiles, can develop predictive models to estimate disease progression and anticipate future functional decline. These models assist in providing personalized prognostic information, optimizing treatment plans, and enabling timely interventions to slow disease progression and improve patient outcomes.

12.5 Data-Driven Research and Drug Development

The integration of AI and IoT facilitates large-scale data collection and analysis, enabling data-driven research and accelerating drug development in neurodegenerative diseases. AI algorithms can analyze genomic data, molecular pathways, and protein–protein interactions to identify potential therapeutic targets and develop precision medicine approaches. This contributes to the discovery of novel treatments and personalized interventions.

12.6 Caregiver Support and Assistance

AI and IoT technologies provide support and assistance to caregivers of individuals with neurodegenerative diseases. Remote monitoring and smart home technology can help caregivers remotely monitor their loved ones' health, receive alerts for emergencies or changes in condition, and access resources and support. This reduces caregiver stress and improves the overall caregiving experience.

12.7 Population Health Management

The integration of AI and IoT enables population-level analysis of neurodegenerative diseases. Aggregated data from diverse sources, combined with AI algorithms and data analytics, can provide valuable insights into disease patterns, risk factors, and treatment responses. This information supports population health management, informs public health strategies, and facilitates targeted interventions.

In conclusion, the opportunities provided by AI and IoT in neurodegenerative diseases are vast and transformative. These technologies enable early detection, personalized treatment, continuous monitoring, remote care, predictive analytics, data-driven research, caregiver support, and population health management. Leveraging the power of AI and IoT has the potential to revolutionize disease management, improve patient outcomes, and enhance the overall quality of life for individuals affected by neurodegenerative diseases.

13 Challenges Faced by AI and IoT in the Field of Neurodegenerative Diseases

13.1 Data Quality and Accessibility

One of the primary challenges in leveraging AI and IoT in neurodegenerative diseases is the availability of high-quality and diverse datasets. Neurodegenerative diseases involve complex and heterogeneous data, including medical imaging, genomics, clinical records, and sensor data. Obtaining comprehensive and standardized datasets that encompass different stages and subtypes of neurodegenerative diseases can be challenging [13]. Variations in data collection methods, privacy concerns, and data silos across healthcare systems can hinder data accessibility and quality. Addressing these challenges requires efforts to harmonize data collection processes, develop interoperable systems, and ensure data privacy and security.

13.2 Ethical Considerations and Privacy

The use of AI and IoT in neurodegenerative diseases raises ethical concerns related to patient privacy, data security, and informed consent. Neurodegenerative diseases involve sensitive health information, and protecting patient confidentiality becomes paramount. IoT devices capture real-time personal health data, and AI algorithms process and analyze this data to derive meaningful insights. Ensuring robust data security measures, anonymization techniques, and adherence to privacy regulations are essential to maintain patient trust. Ethical considerations also include obtaining informed consent from patients and ensuring transparency in how their data is used and shared.

13.3 Technical Complexity and Integration

Implementing AI and IoT technologies in healthcare settings requires expertise in data science, AI algorithms, and IoT infrastructure. Healthcare organizations may face challenges in acquiring and maintaining the necessary technical skills, integrating diverse data sources, and ensuring the interoperability of various IoT devices and platforms. The integration of data from multiple sources, such as electronic health records, wearable devices, and home monitoring systems, can be complex. Overcoming technical challenges requires collaboration between healthcare providers, technology experts, and researchers to develop standardized protocols, implement interoperable systems, and address data integration issues.

13.4 Interpreting and Validating AI Models

AI algorithms, particularly deep learning models, can be complex and operate as "black boxes," making it challenging to interpret the reasoning behind their predictions. Validating the accuracy, reliability, and generalizability of AI models specific to neurodegenerative diseases requires large and diverse datasets, rigorous testing, and validation studies. The lack of interpretability may raise concerns among healthcare professionals who rely on understandable and transparent decision-making processes. Efforts are needed to develop explainable AI models and establish rigorous validation frameworks specific to neurodegenerative diseases.

13.5 User Acceptance and Adoption

The successful implementation of AI and IoT technologies in neurodegenerative diseases depends on user acceptance and adoption. Healthcare professionals, patients, and caregivers may require training, education, and support to understand and effectively utilize these technologies. Resistance to change, lack of familiarity, and concerns about technology reliability and usability can hinder adoption. It is crucial to involve end-users in the design and development of AI and IoT solutions, ensure user-friendly interfaces, address concerns about technology reliability and data security, and demonstrate the value and benefits of AI and IoT in improving patient care.

13.6 Regulatory and Legal Frameworks

The rapid advancements in AI and IoT technologies necessitate regulatory frameworks that keep pace with innovation. Establishing clear guidelines and regulations surrounding the development, deployment, and use of AI and IoT in healthcare, while ensuring patient safety and ethical considerations, is crucial [14]. The lack of harmonized regulations and standards specific to AI and IoT in neurodegenerative diseases can create uncertainty and regulatory challenges.

13.7 Cost and Infrastructure

Implementing AI and IoT technologies may require significant financial investments in infrastructure, including IoT devices, data storage, computational resources, and integration with existing healthcare systems. Healthcare organizations, particularly those with limited resources, may face financial constraints in adopting and maintaining these technologies. Identifying cost-effective solutions, exploring public–private partnerships, and seeking funding opportunities are essential to overcome these challenges. Additionally, the scalability and sustainability of AI and IoT implementations in neurodegenerative diseases need to be carefully considered to ensure long-term viability.

In conclusion, while AI and IoT offer tremendous potential in neurodegenerative diseases, challenges related to data quality and accessibility, ethical considerations, technical complexity and integration, interpretation of AI models, user acceptance, regulatory frameworks, and cost and infrastructure need to be addressed. Overcoming these challenges requires collaborative efforts from healthcare providers, technology experts, policymakers, and regulatory bodies to ensure the responsible and effective implementation of AI and IoT, ultimately improving patient care and advancing research in neurodegenerative diseases.

14 Neural Networks Used in Ai Applications

In the field of neurodegenerative diseases, several types of neural networks are used in AI applications. Here are some networks commonly employed in AI for neurodegenerative diseases:

14.1 Convolutional Neural Networks (CNN)

CNNs are widely used for the analysis of medical imaging data, including magnetic resonance imaging (MRI), positron emission tomography (PET), and computed tomography (CT) scans. CNNs excel at automatically learning relevant features from these images, aiding in tasks such as disease detection, classification, and segmentation.

14.2 Recurrent Neural Networks (RNN)

RNNs are effective for processing sequential data, making them suitable for time series analysis in neurodegenerative diseases. RNNs can model temporal dependencies and have been employed in tasks such as disease progression prediction, speech analysis, and natural language processing for analyzing clinical notes and patient records.

14.3 Long Short-Term Memory (LSTM) Networks

LSTMs, a type of RNN, are designed to capture long-term dependencies in sequential data [15]. They have been utilized in neurodegenerative diseases for tasks like predicting disease progression, analyzing electroencephalography (EEG) signals, and detecting abnormalities in brain wave patterns.

14.4 Generative Adversarial Networks (GAN)

GANs have been explored in neurodegenerative diseases for tasks such as generating synthetic brain images, enhancing low-resolution images, and data augmentation. GANs offer potential in generating realistic and diverse medical images, facilitating training and analysis.

14.5 Autoencoders

Autoencoders are used in neurodegenerative diseases for tasks like anomaly detection, denoising, and feature extraction. By learning a compressed representation of the input data, autoencoders can help identify subtle patterns, detect outliers, and reduce the dimensionality of high-dimensional data [16].

14.6 Deep Reinforcement Learning (DRL)

DRL combines deep learning with reinforcement learning principles. In neurodegenerative diseases, DRL has been explored in areas such as personalized treatment optimization, adaptive therapy planning, and clinical decision-making to maximize long-term patient outcomes.

It's important to note that the choice of network architecture depends on the specific task, available data, and research goals in the context of neurodegenerative diseases. Researchers continually explore and develop novel network architectures and hybrid models to address the unique challenges and requirements of this field [17].

15 Conclusion

The integration of AI and the IoT in the field of neurodegenerative diseases holds immense promise for revolutionizing disease management, improving patient care, and advancing research efforts. Through AI and IoT technologies, healthcare professionals and researchers can harness the power of data-driven insights, real-time monitoring, and personalized interventions to enhance early detection, diagnosis, treatment, and overall quality of life for individuals affected by neurodegenerative diseases. AI algorithms, such as machine learning and deep learning models, have demonstrated remarkable capabilities in neurodegenerative disease research. They can analyze complex and heterogeneous data sources, including medical imaging, genomic profiles, and clinical records, to uncover valuable patterns, identify biomarkers, and predict disease progression. These models aid in early detection, accurate diagnosis, and personalized treatment planning, facilitating timely interventions and improved patient outcomes. Furthermore, AI-driven analysis of medical imaging data has proven invaluable in identifying disease-related patterns, enabling more precise and efficient disease detection and monitoring. The IoT plays a vital role in the context of neurodegenerative diseases by enabling continuous remote monitoring and real-time data collection. Wearable devices, smart home technology, and telemedicine platforms equipped with IoT capabilities provide a wealth of patient-generated data, including vital signs, movement patterns, and activities of daily living. This real-time data empowers healthcare professionals to remotely monitor patients, intervene proactively, and optimize treatment plans based on personalized insights. Moreover, IoT-enabled devices enhance patient engagement and self-management by promoting adherence to medication regimens, facilitating remote consultations, and supporting the overall well-being of individuals living with neurodegenerative diseases. The combination of AI and IoT technologies also opens up new possibilities for predictive analytics, population health management, and data-driven research. By leveraging AI algorithms and big data analytics, healthcare providers and researchers can identify disease patterns, predict disease outcomes, and assess treatment responses on a population level. This information is invaluable for informing public health strategies, optimizing healthcare resource allocation, and identifying potential targets for drug development. In conclusion, the integration of AI and IoT in neurodegenerative diseases offers transformative opportunities to advance diagnosis, treatment, monitoring, and overall patient care. These technologies empower healthcare professionals with data-driven insights, facilitate remote monitoring and personalized interventions, and enable collaborative research efforts. However, addressing challenges related to data quality, privacy, technical complexity, user acceptance, regulations, and cost is crucial for realizing the full potential of AI and IoT in neurodegenerative diseases. By overcoming these challenges and harnessing the power of AI and IoT, we can improve the lives of individuals affected by neurodegenerative diseases, enhance disease management, and accelerate the discovery of innovative therapies.

16 Future Work

The demand for novel strategies to enhance diagnosis, therapy, and overall care is expanding as the prevalence of neurodegenerative disorders rises. Unprecedented prospects in the study of neurodegenerative disorders are now available thanks to the convergence of AI and the IoT in recent years. The connectivity provided by IoT devices and the data processing capabilities of AI have enabled new applications that have revolutionized disease monitoring, personalized therapies, and research developments. This study intends to investigate the synergistic impacts of AI and IoT on neurodegenerative disorders, highlighting the exciting future these technologies have in the battle against these crippling conditions. By tapping into the potential of AI algorithms and the interconnectedness of IoT, healthcare experts and researchers can uncover fresh insights, enhance patient well-being, and pave the path for more precise and impactful interventions. As AI and IoT technologies make progress, it becomes essential to tackle the moral considerations linked to their application in neurodegenerative illnesses. Upcoming studies can delve into ethical frameworks, policy recommendations, and oversight mechanisms that ensure the responsible and moral use of AI and IoT solutions. This encompasses dealing with concerns related to safeguarding data privacy, obtaining informed consent, addressing algorithmic biases, and ensuring fair distribution of technological advantages. Through the development of thorough ethical guidelines, researchers and healthcare practitioners can navigate the ethical dilemmas associated with AI and IoT in neurodegenerative diseases, thus fostering public confidence in these innovations. In conclusion, future studies concerning AI and IoT in diseases that affect the brain could center on bringing together different types of data, making real-time monitoring and intervention systems even better, helping AI models make more sense, looking at data over a long period of time, checking out how augmented and virtual reality could help, encouraging everyone to share data, and dealing with what's right and fair. These research areas could really make AI and IoT even more helpful for managing brain-related diseases. This could mean better outcomes for patients and more personalized ways to treat them. If we keep researching and coming up with new ideas in these areas, we could see big changes in how we care for people with brain-related diseases.

References

1. Bosch, J., Olsson, H. H., Brinne, B., & Crnkovic, I. (2022). AI engineering: Realizing the potential of AI. *IEEE Software, 39*(6), 23–27. https://doi.org/10.1109/ms.2022.3199621
2. Xin, J. Z. (2021). Neurodegenerative diseases and their related treatment. *E3s Web of Conferences, 271*, 3020–3020. https://doi.org/10.1051/e3sconf/202127103020
3. Lewis, P. R., Marsh, S., & Pitt, J. (2021). AI vs "AI": Synthetic minds or speech acts. *IEEE Technology and Society Magazine, 40*, 6–13. https://doi.org/10.1109/mts.2021.3077052
4. Sponner, M., Waschneck, B., Kumar, A. (2022). AI-driven performance modeling for AI inference workloads. *Electronics, 11*(15), 2316–2316. https://doi.org/10.3390/electronics11152316
5. Mathur, S., & Arora, A. IoT and PKI based security architecture.
6. Leake, D. B. (2012). The diversity of AI. *AI Magazine, 33*(1), 9–9. https://doi.org/10.1609/aimag.v33i1.2404
7. Husain, M. (2021). Sleep and neurodegenerative diseases. *Brain, 144*(3), 695–696. https://doi.org/10.1093/brain/awab031
8. Mortada, I., Farah, R., Nabha, S., Ojcius, D. M., Fares, Y., Almawi, W. Y., & Sadier, N. S. (2021). Immunotherapies for neurodegenerative diseases. *Frontiers in Neurology, 12.* https://doi.org/10.3389/fneur.2021.654739
9. Ruz, C., Alcantud, J. L., Montero, F., Duran, R., & Bandres-Ciga, S. (2020). Proteotoxicity and neurodegenerative diseases. *International Journal of Molecular Sciences, 21*(16), 5646–5646. https://doi.org/10.3390/ijms21165646
10. Don Monroe, V. (2022). Accelerating AI. *Communications of the ACM, 65*(3), 15–16. https://doi.org/10.1145/3510554
11. Mikhalskii, A. I., & Novoseltseva, J. A. (2018). Application of data analysis methods in research of neurodegenerative diseases. In *2018 eleventh international conference "Management of large-scale system development"* MLSD (pp. 1–4). IEEE.
12. Migliore, L. U. C. I. A., Fontana, I., Colognato, R., Coppede, F. A. B. I. O., Siciliano, G. A. B. R. I. E. L. E., & Murri, L. U. I. G. I. (2005). Searching for the role and the most suitable biomarkers of oxidative stress in Alzheimer's disease and other neurodegenerative diseases. *Neurobiology of Aging, 26*(5), 587–595.
13. Mathur, S., Singla, T., Bharat, K., & Rana, A. (2022). AIIOT: Emerging IoT with AI technologies. *A Fusion of AI and IoT for Emerging Cyber Systems*, 269–291.
14. Mathur, S., & Datta, K. (2021). Prediction of Covid-19 cases in India through machine learning using Python. In *2021 9th international conference on reliability, Infocom technologies and optimization (trends and future directions) (ICRITO)* (pp. 1–6). IEEE.

15. Mathur, S. (2021). Evolving IoT and green IoT in healthcare perspective. *Evolving Role of AI and IoMT in the Healthcare Market*, 175–197.
16. Shusharina, N., Yukhnenko, D., Botman, S., Sapunov, V., Savinov, V., Kamyshov, G., & Voznyuk, I. (2023). Modern methods of diagnostics and treatment of neurodegenerative diseases and depression. *Diagnostics, 13*(3), 573.
17. Mathur, S. (2022). Modeling the stubble burning generated airborne contamination with air pollution components through MATLAB. *Earth Science Informatics, 15*(2), 1137-1146.

Explainable Artificial Intelligence (XAI) on Neurogenerative Diseases

Loveleen Gaur and Devanshi Gaur

Abstract Artificial intelligence (AI) has the potential to revolutionize our understanding, diagnosis, and treatment of neurodegenerative diseases. Neurodegenerative diseases, such as Alzheimer's disease, Parkinson's disease, and Huntington's disease, are characterized by the progressive loss of structure and function of neurons in the brain. AI has the potential to make significant contributions to the understanding, diagnosis, and treatment of neurodegenerative diseases. By leveraging its capabilities in data analysis, pattern recognition, and predictive modeling, AI can accelerate research, improve patient outcomes, and ultimately help in finding effective treatments for these debilitating conditions. Explainable AI(XAI) refers to artificial intelligence systems that can explain their reasoning and decisions to humans in a transparent and understandable way. As AI systems become more complex, being able to understand how they arrive at conclusions is important for building trust and ensuring the systems make fair and accurate decisions.

Keywords Explainable artificial intelligence · Neurodegenerative diseases · Advancements in neuroimaging

1 Introduction

XAI is a subfield of artificial intelligence that focuses on developing techniques and methods to make the decision-making process of AI models interpretable, transparent, and understandable to humans. This is especially critical in areas like healthcare, where understanding the reasoning behind a diagnosis or prediction can impact patient outcomes and physician decisions [1].

L. Gaur (✉)
Taylor's University, Subang Jaya, Malaysia
e-mail: gaurloveleen@yahoo.com

D. Gaur
Florida International University, Miami, FL, USA
e-mail: dgaur002@fiu.edu

© The Author(s), under exclusive license to Springer Nature Switzerland AG 2024

L. Gaur et al. (eds.), *AI and Neuro-Degenerative Diseases*, Studies in Computational Intelligence 1131, https://doi.org/10.1007/978-3-031-53148-4_3

Neurodegenerative diseases, such as Alzheimer's, Parkinson's, and Huntington's diseases, are conditions characterized by the progressive degeneration or death of nerve cells (neurons). The intricate biological processes underlying these diseases, combined with the high variability in patient symptoms and disease progression, make them a complex challenge for both diagnosis and treatment.

The emerging field of XAI holds great promise for unlocking new insights into the mechanisms and treatment of neurodegenerative diseases like Alzheimer's, Parkinson's, and ALS. XAI refers to AI systems that can explain their internal reasoning and decision-making processes to human users in a transparent and understandable way. As machine learning algorithms become more complex, being able to interpret their workings is critical. In neurodegenerative disease, XAI could analyze MRI, PET, and other medical scan data to identify imaging biomarkers indicative of disease progression. It could highlight the regions of interest and patterns in the data justifying its assessments. This allows clinicians to validate the system's conclusions. XAI systems could also analyze large and complex molecular, genomic, and clinical datasets to discover new prognostic biomarkers. The AI would provide explanations for the key relationships and data features driving the discovery of a new biomarker. On the treatment side, XAI could take a patient's specific profile and data and provide personalized predictions for disease trajectory and optimal therapies. The system would explain the underlying rationale which doctors could then evaluate. XAI offers the promise of powerful AI systems that can lend transparency to their insights. However, work is still needed to develop XAI that is accurate, consistent, and informative in the context of the complexity of neurodegenerative diseases [2–5].

2 Role of XAI in Neurogenerative Diseases

Here's how XAI can contribute to understand and address neurodegenerative diseases:

- **Diagnostic Aid**: Machine learning models can analyze vast amounts of medical data, such as brain scans, to identify early signs of neurodegenerative diseases. However, clinicians need to understand the rationale behind such diagnoses. XAI can help visualize which specific features or regions of a brain scan contributed most to a particular diagnosis, aiding clinicians in making informed decisions [6].
- **Treatment Personalization**: By analyzing patient data and making the decision-making process transparent, XAI models can suggest personalized treatment plans. Doctors can see the reasons behind suggested treatments and can choose interventions tailored to individual patient needs[7].
- **Biomarker Discovery**: AI models can help in the identification of new biomarkers for neurodegenerative diseases by sifting through massive datasets. XAI can then provide insights into why these biomarkers are relevant, allowing researchers to better understand disease mechanisms.

- **Drug Development**: By understanding which features or biological markers an AI model deems significant, researchers can potentially discover new therapeutic targets for drug development. XAI ensures that these insights are not just a black-box prediction but are backed by interpretable reasoning.
- **Patient and Caregiver Support**: Transparent AI models can provide clearer explanations to patients and caregivers about disease progression and treatment rationales. This can improve patient trust and adherence to treatment.
- **Research Insights**: As researchers attempt to unravel the mysteries of neurodegenerative diseases, XAI can assist by highlighting potential areas of interest or patterns that may not be immediately evident to human researchers.
- **Regulatory and Ethical Decisions**: When AI is used in healthcare, there's a need for transparency for regulatory approvals and ethical considerations. XAI ensures that decisions made by the model can be understood, reviewed, and critiqued by human experts [8–10].

Incorporating XAI in the domain of neurodegenerative diseases has the potential to bridge the gap between advanced machine learning models and their real-world clinical applications. It fosters trust, drives research, and, most importantly, can enhance patient care and outcomes by offering clear insights into the otherwise opaque decision-making processes of AI.

3 XAI Techniques for Neurodegenerative Diseases

When applying Explainable AI (XAI) techniques to neurodegenerative diseases, the methods primarily hinge on the type of data being analyzed and the model being used [11, 12] The following is an overview of some widely used XAI techniques, specifically tailored to the domain of neurodegenerative diseases:

- *Feature Importance Visualization*: It displays the significance of input features on a model's predictions. It aids understanding by ranking and visually depicting the impact of each feature, helping users interpret model behavior and decisions, promoting transparency and trust in AI systems. The application is for datasets that contain patient information, clinical measures, genetic markers, and other tabular data. Tools like SHAP (SHapley Additive exPlanations) or LIME (Local Interpretable Model-agnostic Explanations) can be used to illustrate which features (e.g., specific genes or clinical measures) were most influential in each prediction [13].
- *Attention Mechanisms in Neural Networks*: It enhances interpretability by highlighting input elements affecting predictions. It improves transparency by assigning varying weights to inputs, allowing users to comprehend model decisions, and fostering trust in complex AI systems. The application is primarily for deep learning models analyzing sequential data or when using architectures like transformers. In this technique, the attention weights can be visualized to show which parts of the input data the model paid most attention to when deciding.

- *Activation Maximization*: It optimizes input data to evoke desired neuron activations. This aids model comprehension by generating inputs that trigger specific features, contributing to transparency and insight into neural network behavior, thus enhancing trust in AI systems. The application is for image data, such as MRI or PET scans. This method visualizes what a particular neuron in a deep learning model "prefers to see" by adjusting the input image to maximize the activation of that neuron.
- *Grad-CAM (Gradient-weighted Class Activation Mapping)*: It identifies important image regions influencing neural network predictions. By visualizing gradient-based heatmaps, it enhances interpretability, highlighting regions crucial for predictions and enabling users to understand model decisions, bolstering transparency and trust in AI. The application is for convolutional neural networks (CNNs) analyzing neuroimaging data. In this technique it visualizes the regions in the image that were most important for the model's decision, providing a heatmap overlay on the original image [14–16].
- *Counterfactual Explanations*: It creates alternate instances to clarify model decisions. By showing how small changes lead to different outcomes, they enhance understanding, making AI systems transparent. This fosters trust and comprehension of complex models, promoting responsible and accountable AI deployment. The application is for patient profiles and clinical data. It explains model decisions by showing how the input data would have to change to alter the model's prediction. For instance, it can show how certain clinical measures would need to change to shift a patient from a "high risk" to a "low risk" category.
- *Feature Interaction Visualization*: It illustrates how input features collaboratively influence model predictions. By displaying dependencies and interactions, it aids users in comprehending intricate relationships, enhancing transparency and confidence in AI systems' decision-making processes. The application is for high-dimensional data where interactions between features could be significant. Tools like SHAP can also show how features interact with one another to influence a model's decision.
- *Rule Extraction*: It distills interpretable rules from complex models. By converting intricate behaviors into understandable if–then statements, it enables users to grasp decision logic, promoting transparency and trust while maintaining the model's predictive power and performance. The application is for decision trees or simpler models analyzing patient data. The technique is to convert the model's logic into a set of human-readable rules. Techniques like BRL (Bayesian Rule Lists) can be particularly useful.
- *Model Simplification*: is a process in which complex machine learning models are transformed into more interpretable and computationally efficient versions. This aids in enhancing transparency, reducing computational resources, and facilitating easier deployment, all while preserving the core predictive capabilities of the original model. The technique is to train a more interpretable model, like a linear regression or decision tree, to approximate the predictions of a complex model.

- *Prototype Selection*: Prototype selection is a data reduction technique that chooses a subset of representative instances from a dataset. It reduces computational complexity, storage requirements, and noise while preserving essential information. This aids in streamlining machine learning tasks, improving model efficiency, and accelerating decision-making processes. The application is for clustering or understanding patient subgroups. The technique is to identify prototype instances that represent clusters within the data. This can help in understanding the "typical" characteristics of certain patient groups.

When choosing an XAI technique for neurodegenerative diseases, it's crucial to consider the clinical context, the stakeholders involved (e.g., clinicians, patients, caregivers), and the type of data and models in use. An approach that integrates multiple techniques can often provide more comprehensive insights and enhance the trustworthiness of AI-driven analyses [17–20].

4 Applications of XAI in Neurodegenerative Diseases

Here are some innovative and mind-blowing applications of XAI in the context of neurodegenerative diseases:

- *Early Disease Detection through Voice Analysis*: XAI could be used to develop AI models that analyze subtle changes in speech patterns and voice characteristics. These models could detect early signs of neurodegenerative diseases like Parkinson's or Alzheimer's, potentially enabling non-invasive and cost-effective early diagnosis.
- *Neuroimaging Interpretation*: XAI could help neuroimaging specialists and researchers understand the complex patterns in brain images that are associated with neurodegenerative diseases. This could lead to more accurate diagnosis and prediction of disease progression by highlighting regions of interest and their significance.
- *Real-time Symptom Prediction*: AI models combined with XAI could continuously analyze a patient's health data, such as movement patterns, heart rate variability, and cognitive performance. The models could provide real-time predictions of symptom exacerbations in conditions like ALS, enabling timely interventions.
- *Personalized Treatment Recommendations*: XAI-powered AI models could analyze a patient's medical history, genetic makeup, and response to treatments. This information could then be used to provide personalized treatment recommendations that consider the patient's unique characteristics and the likely effectiveness of different interventions.
- *Brain-Computer Interfaces (BCIs) Interpretation*: XAI could be used to translate the output of BCIs, which allow communication between the brain and external devices. This could assist individuals with severe neurodegenerative diseases, like ALS, to convey their thoughts and intentions more effectively.

- *Predictive Modeling for Disease Progression*: XAI could enhance predictive models that estimate disease progression trajectories. By explaining the factors contributing to predictions, clinicians and researchers could better understand the disease's complexity and potentially identify novel intervention opportunities.
- *Virtual Reality (VR) Therapy Enhancement*: XAI could optimize VR-based therapy for neurodegenerative patients. The AI could adjust the therapy environment and scenarios based on real-time monitoring and understanding of the patient's cognitive and emotional states.
- *Neurological Data Artifacts Identification*: XAI could automatically detect and explain artifacts in neurological data, such as EEG or fMRI signals. This could improve the accuracy of data interpretation and the reliability of insights drawn from these data sources.
- *Brain Network Analysis*: XAI could unravel the intricate connections between different brain regions and their role in disease development. This could provide breakthrough insights into how neurodegenerative diseases spread within the brain and influence cognitive functions.
- *Lifestyle Intervention Recommendations*: AI models powered by XAI could analyze a patient's lifestyle habits, such as diet, exercise, and sleep patterns. By explaining how these factors contribute to disease risk or progression, patients could receive tailored recommendations for lifestyle modifications.
- *AI-Aided Drug Design for Neurodegeneration*: XAI could assist in the design of novel drugs by explaining how specific molecular interactions influence neurodegenerative processes. This could accelerate drug discovery efforts by providing more transparent insights into potential therapeutic targets.

These mind-blowing applications of XAI have the potential to revolutionize our understanding, diagnosis, treatment, and management of neurodegenerative diseases, leading to improved patient outcomes and enhancing our overall capabilities in neurology and neuroscience [21–25].

5 Future Perspectives and Opportunities

Explainable Artificial Intelligence (XAI) techniques offer significant future perspectives and opportunities in the field of neurodegenerative diseases, such as Alzheimer's disease, Parkinson's disease, and Amyotrophic Lateral Sclerosis (ALS). Here's a detailed exploration of these possibilities:

- *Early Detection and Diagnosis*: XAI models can analyze diverse data sources, including medical imaging, genomics, and clinical records, to identify subtle patterns and biomarkers indicative of neurodegenerative diseases. By providing interpretable insights, XAI can assist in early detection, enabling timely interventions and improved patient outcomes.

- *Predictive Modeling*: XAI can develop predictive models that forecast disease progression and risk factors. These models can help clinicians and caregivers anticipate patient needs, personalize treatment plans, and allocate resources efficiently, ultimately enhancing patient care and reducing healthcare costs.
- *Treatment Personalization*: XAI can aid in tailoring treatment plans for individual patients. By analyzing patient data, including genetic profiles and responses to therapies, XAI can recommend the most effective treatments, dosages, and interventions, minimizing adverse effects and optimizing therapeutic outcomes.
- *Drug Discovery*: XAI can accelerate drug discovery by identifying potential drug candidates and predicting their efficacy in targeting specific disease mechanisms. This can lead to the development of more effective treatments and reduce the time and costs associated with drug development.
- *Neuroimaging Analysis*: XAI can enhance the analysis of neuroimaging data, such as MRI and PET scans. It can highlight regions of interest, track disease progression, and provide insights into structural and functional changes in the brain, aiding researchers and clinicians in understanding the disease's underlying mechanisms.
- *Interpretability in Black-Box Models*: Many deep learning models used in healthcare are considered black boxes due to their complexity. XAI techniques, like attention maps and feature importance visualization, can provide interpretable explanations for these models' predictions, increasing trust and acceptance among clinicians and patients.
- *Data Integration*: Neurodegenerative diseases involve complex interactions between genetic, environmental, and clinical factors. XAI can integrate data from various sources and identify meaningful connections between these factors, facilitating a holistic understanding of disease etiology and progression.
- *Continuous Monitoring and Disease Management*: XAI-powered wearable devices and remote monitoring systems can continuously collect patient data, allowing for real-time disease monitoring and management. Any deviations from baseline can trigger alerts, enabling timely interventions and reducing hospitalizations.

Ethical and Regulatory Considerations

- As XAI techniques become more integrated into healthcare, addressing ethical concerns, data privacy, and regulatory compliance will be crucial. Developing transparent and ethical AI solutions will be essential to gain public trust and ensure responsible use.
- *Collaboration and Knowledge Sharing*: Collaboration between AI researchers, medical professionals, and data scientists will be vital to harness the full potential of XAI in neurodegenerative diseases. Sharing knowledge and best practices will accelerate progress and improve patient care.

Future perspectives and opportunities for eXplainable Artificial Intelligence (XAI) in neurodegenerative diseases are promising. XAI can help decipher the complex mechanisms of diseases like Alzheimer's and Parkinson's by providing interpretable insights into neural network behavior. This can lead to earlier diagnosis, more targeted treatments, and a deeper understanding of disease progression. Additionally, XAI can facilitate personalized medicine approaches, enabling tailored interventions based on individual patient data. Collaborations between AI researchers, medical professionals, and data scientists are crucial to harness the full potential of XAI in addressing the challenges of neurodegenerative diseases. Ethical considerations, data privacy, and regulatory compliance will also be key areas of focus in this evolving field. Overall, XAI holds great potential to revolutionize our understanding and management of neurodegenerative diseases in the coming years [26–28].

6 Conclusion

XAI techniques hold immense promise in advancing our understanding, diagnosis, and treatment of neurodegenerative diseases. These techniques can empower healthcare professionals with interpretable insights, enable personalized medicine, expedite drug discovery, and enhance overall patient care. However, addressing ethical, regulatory, and data privacy concerns is essential to ensure that XAI is used responsibly and effectively in this critical area of healthcare.

References

1. Duong, M. T., Rauschecker, A. M., & Mohan, S. (2020). Diverse applications of artificial intelligence in neuroradiology. *Neuroimaging Clinical of North American, 30*(4), 505–516. https://doi.org/10.1016/j.nic.2020.07.003. Epub 2020 Sep 17. PMID: 33039000; PMCID: PMC8530432.
2. Bhandari, M., Neupane, A., Mallik, S., Gaur, L., & Qin, H. (2023). Auguring fake face images using dual input convolution neural network. *Journal of Imaging, 9*(1), 3. https://doi.org/10.3390/jimaging9010003
3. Gaur, L., & Sahoo, B. M. (2022). Introduction to explainable AI and intelligent transportation. In *Explainable Artificial Intelligence for Intelligent Transportation Systems*. Springer, Cham. https://doi.org/10.1007/978-3-031-09644-0_1.
4. Ross, C. A., & Poirier, M. A. (2004). Protein aggregation and neurodegenerative disease. *Nature Medicine, 10*(Suppl), S10–S17. https://doi.org/10.1038/nm1066
5. Glass, C. K., Saijo, K., Winner, B., Marchetto, M. C., & Gage, F. H. (2010). Mechanisms underlying inflammation in neurodegeneration. *Cell, 140*, 918–934. https://doi.org/10.1016/j.cell.2010.02.016
6. Dias, V., Junn, E., & Mouradian, M. M. (2013). The role of oxidative stress in Parkinson's disease. *Journal of Parkinson's Disease, 3*, 461–491. https://doi.org/10.3233/JPD-130230
7. Shortliffe, E. H., & Buchanan, B. G. (1975). A model of inexact reasoning in medicine. *Mathematical Biosciences, 23*, 351–379. https://doi.org/10.1016/0025-5564(75)90047-4.
8. Lindsay, R. K., Buchanan, B. G., Feigenbaum, E. A., & Lederberg, J. (1993). DENDRAL: A case study of the first expert system for scientific hypothesis formation. *Artificial Intelligent, 61*, 209–261. https://doi.org/10.1016/0004-3702(93)90068-M.

9. Miller, R. A., Pople, H. E. J., & Myers, J. D. (1982). Internist-1, an experimental computer-based diagnostic consultant for general internal medicine. *New England Journal of Medicine, 307*, 468–476. https://doi.org/10.1056/NEJM198208193070803
10. de Dombal, F. T., Leaper, D. J., Staniland, J. R., McCann, A. P., & Horrocks, J. C. (1972). Computer-aided diagnosis of acute abdominal pain. *British Medical Journal, 2*, 9 LP–13. https://doi.org/10.1136/bmj.2.5804.9.
11. Ghose, P., Alavi, M., Tabassum, M., Ashraf Uddin, M., Biswas, M., Mahbub, K., Gaur, L., Mallik, S., & Zhao, Z. (2022). Detecting COVID-19 infection status from chest X-ray and CT scan via single transfer learning-driven approach. *Frontiers in Genetics, 13*, 980338. https://doi.org/10.3389/fgene.2022.980338
12. Gaur, L., Bhandari, M., Razdan, T., Mallik, S., & Zhao, Z. (2022). Explanation-driven deep learning model for prediction of brain tumour status using MRI image data. *Frontiers in Genetics, 13*, 822666. https://doi.org/10.3389/fgene.2022.822666
13. De Fauw, J., Ledsam, J. R., Romera-Paredes, B., Nikolov, S., Tomasev, N., Blackwell, S., Askham, H., Glorot, X., O'Donoghue, B., Visentin, D., van den Driessche, G., Lakshminarayanan, B., Meyer, C., Mackinder, F., Bouton, S., Ayoub, K., Chopra, R., King, D., Karthikesalingam, A., … Ronneberger, O. (2018). Clinically applicable deep learning for diagnosis and referral in retinal disease. *Nature Medicine, 24*, 1342–1350. https://doi.org/10.1038/s41591-018-0107-6
14. Bhandari, M., Parajuli, P., Chapagain, P., & Gaur, L. (2022). Evaluating performance of Adam optimization by proposing energy index. In K. Santosh, R. Hegadi, U. Pal (eds), *Recent Trends in Image Processing and Pattern Recognition*. RTIP2R 2021. Communications in Computer and Information Science, vol. 1576. Springer, Cham. https://doi.org/10.1007/978-3-031-07005-1_15
15. Raghupathi, W., & Raghupathi, V. (2014). Big data analytics in healthcare: Promise and potential. *Health Information Science System, 2*, 3. https://doi.org/10.1186/2047-2501-2-3
16. Gaur, L., Bhatia, U., Jhanjhi, N. Z., et al. (2023). Medical image-based detection of COVID-19 using deep convolution neural networks. *Multimedia Systems, 29*, 1729–1738. https://doi.org/10.1007/s00530-021-00794-6
17. Alzubaidi, L., Zhang, J., Humaidi, A.J., Al-Dujaili, A., Duan, Y., Al-Shamma, O., Santamaría, J., Fadhel, M.A., Al-Amidie, M., & Farhan, L. (2021). *Review of deep learning: Concepts, CNN architectures, challenges, applications, future directions*. Springer International Publishing.https://doi.org/10.1186/s40537-021-00444-8
18. Pyrros, A., Rodriguez Fernandez, J., Borstelmann, S. M., Flanders, A., Wenzke, D., Hart, E., Horowitz, J. M., Nikolaidis, P., Willis, M., Chen, A., Cole, P., Siddiqui, N., Muzaffar, M., Muzaffar, N., McVean, J., Menchaca, M., Katsaggelos, A. K., Koyejo, S., & Galanter, W. (2022). Validation of a deep learning, value-based care model to predict mortality and comorbidities from chest radiographs in COVID-19. *PLOS Digital Health, 1*, e0000057. https://doi.org/10.1371/journal.pdig.0000057
19. Wang, L., Li, P., Hou, M., Zhang, X., Cao, X., & Li, H. (2021). Construction of a risk prediction model for Alzheimer's disease in the elderly population. *BMC Neurology, 21*, 271. https://doi.org/10.1186/s12883-021-02276-8
20. Gaur, L., Singh, G., & Agarwal, V. (2021). Leveraging artificial intelligence tools to combat the COVID-19 crisis. In P. K. Singh, G. Veselov, V. Vyatkin, A. Pljonkin, J. M. Dodero, & Y. Kumar (eds) *Futuristic Trends in Network and Communication Technologies*. FTNCT 2020. Communications in Computer and Information Science, vol. 1395. Springer, Singapore. https://doi.org/10.1007/978-981-16-1480-4_28
21. Sweeney, L. (2002). K-Anonymity: A model for protecting privacy. *International Journal Uncertain. Fuzziness Knowledge-Based System, 10*, 557–570. https://doi.org/10.1142/S0218488502001648.
22. Saeed, S., Haroon, H. B., Naqvi, M., Jhanjhi, N. Z., Ahmad, M., & Gaur, L. (2022). A systematic mapping study of low-grade Tumor of brain cancer and CSF fluid detecting approaches and parameters. In N. Zaman, L. Gaur, & M. Humayun (Eds.), *Approaches and Applications of*

Deep Learning in Virtual Medical Care (pp. 236–259). IGI Global. https://doi.org/10.4018/978-1-7998-8929-8.ch010

23. Gaur, L., Bhatia, U., & Bakshi, S. (2022). Cloud driven framework for skin cancer detection using deep CNN. *2022 2nd International Conference on Innovative Practices in Technology and Management (ICIPTM)*, Gautam Buddha Nagar, India, pp. 460–464, https://doi.org/10.1109/ICIPTM54933.2022.9754216.
24. Ghose, P., Sharmin, S., Gaur, L., & Zhao, Z. (2022). Grid-search integrated optimized support vector machine model for breast cancer detection. *2022 IEEE International Conference on Bioinformatics and Biomedicine (BIBM)*, Las Vegas, NV, USA, 2022, pp. 2846–2852. https://doi.org/10.1109/BIBM55620.2022.9995703.
25. Gaur, L., Jhanjhi, N. Z., Bakshi, S., & Gupta, P. (2022). Analyzing consequences of artificial intelligence on jobs using topic modeling and keyword extraction. *2022 2nd International Conference on Innovative Practices in Technology and Management (ICIPTM)*, Gautam Buddha Nagar, India, pp. 435–440, https://doi.org/10.1109/ICIPTM54933.2022.9754064.
26. Counts, S. E., Ikonomovic, M. D., Mercado, N., Vega, I. E., & Mufson, E. J. (2017). Biomarkers for the early detection and progression of Alzheimer's disease. *Neurotherapeutics, 14*, 35–53. https://doi.org/10.1007/s13311-016-0481-z
27. Kormas, P., & Moutzouri, A. (2020). Current psychological approaches in neurodegenerative diseases. In P. Vlamos, I. S. Kotsireas & I. Tarnanas (eds.) *Handbook of Computational Neurodegeneration*, pp. 1–29. Springer International Publishing, Cham. https://doi.org/10.1007/978-3-319-75479-6_10-1.
28. Gaur L, Siarry P, Abraham A and Castillo O (2024) Editorial: advancements of deep learning in medical imaging for neurodegenerative diseases. Front Neurosci 18:1361055. https://doi.org/10.3389/fnins.2024.1361055

Clinical Genomics to Drug Discovery Using Machine Learning for Neurodegenerative Disorders: A Future Perspective

Abhishek Kumar Sahu, Rosaleen Sahoo, Lingaraj Jena, Sundeep Singh Saluja, and Parameswar Sahu

Abstract Neurodegenerative diseases affect the central nervous system and lead to death of neuronal cells. Development of therapeutics for neurodegenerative diseases is more challenging as compared to other diseases. Exploring the association of neurodegenerative diseases with human gut microbiome can lead to development of microbiome-based therapeutics. Advancement in tools and techniques has changed the face of traditional clinical genomics. Integration of omics approach with computer-aided drug discovery and artificial intelligence gives a multidimensional insight into diagnosis and prognosis of neurodegenerative diseases. Faecal samples of patients of neurodegenerative diseases can be analysed using Next Generation Sequencing approach and can be further integrate with drug discovery approach to get insight into the important genes of highly abundant microbes in human gut. Furthermore, Magnetic Resonance Imaging (MRI), Single-photon emission computed tomography (SPECT), and positron emission tomography (PET) of

A. K. Sahu
Department of Bioinformatics, Centre for Post Graduate Studies, Odisha University of Agriculture and Technology, Bhubaneswar, Odisha, India

R. Sahoo
Academy of Scientific and Innovative Research (AcSIR), Ghaziabad, Uttar Pradesh, India

Biochemical Science Division, CSIR-National Chemical Laboratory, Pune, Maharashtra, India

L. Jena
Laboratory Oncology Unit, Dr. B.R.A. IRCH, All India Institute of Medical Sciences (AIIMS), New Delhi, India

S. S. Saluja (✉) · P. Sahu (✉)
Central Molecular Laboratory, Govind Ballabh Pant Institute of Post Graduate Medical Education and Research, New Delhi, India
e-mail: sundeepsaluja@yahoo.co.in

P. Sahu
e-mail: bio.parameswar@gmail.com

S. S. Saluja
Department of Gastrointestinal Surgery, Govind Ballabh Pant Institute of Post Graduate Medical Education and Research, New Delhi, India

© The Author(s), under exclusive license to Springer Nature Switzerland AG 2024

L. Gaur et al. (eds.), *AI and Neuro-Degenerative Diseases*, Studies in Computational Intelligence 1131, https://doi.org/10.1007/978-3-031-53148-4_4

patients can be analysed using various Artificial Intelligence approach to develop models for prediction and analysis of the neurodegenerative disease as well as classification of diseases.

1 Introduction

Twenty first century has been a witness of the advancement of science and technology for the last decades. Progress of scientific ideas and application of the improved methodologies in every aspects of human welfare has unlocked the doors of interdisciplinary research for furtherance. Advancement in the field of data science and its' implication in healthcare sector has favoured the clinicians for better diagnostic models and precision medicine. Implementation of artificial intelligence in the direction of clinical genomics has enabled healthcare researchers towards precision medicine. However, a lot of obstacles are yet to be overtaken. Correlation of clinical genomics with drug discovery using artificial intelligence for neurodegenerative disorders has been done further in this book chapter.

2 Neurodegenerative Diseases

Neurodegenerative diseasesoccur commonly in elderly population and show characteristics like decrease in function of sensory system, functional alterations in the central nervous systems and death of nerve cells [12]. Prevalence of common neurodegenerative diseases like Alzheimer's and Parkinson's disease increases with age [16].

The most common neurodegenerative disease is Alzheimer's disease. Cognitive function decreases with the on-set of Alzheimer's disease. Pathology of Alzheimer's disease starts with the deposition of amyloid-beta, followed by the formation of hyperphosphorylated tau protein, which compose plaques and neurofibrillary tangles [8]. It is reported that the deposition of amyloid-beta and tau protein occurs years before the onset of clinical dementia symptoms [22].

Parkinson's disease holds the second position worldwide after Alzheimer's diseaseamong neurodegenerative diseases. Parkinson's disease, a complex diseases characterised by several motor and non-motor symptoms. Non-motor symptomsincludes gastrointestinal dysfunction, sleep disorders, and sensory disturbanceswhich occur before the on-set of motor symptomsand impairs the life of patient [39].

3 Gut Microbes in Neurodegenerative Diseases

Human gut microbiome predominantly comprises of bacterial phyla. Microbes in the human gut produces around ~10^{13}–10^{14} cells, which is larger than the cells produced by human. Likewise, genes expressed by human gut microbe is about 50–100 fold larger than the human genes [21, 31]. Human gut microbiome plays significant role on human health as well asdiseases [3].

It has been reported in many articles that human gut play vital role in etiology of Alzheimer's disease. 16S rRNA based method identified that *Bacteroidetes* and *Firmicutes* are the predominant in adult human gut, whereas the abundance of *Actinobacteria, Proteobacteria* and *Verrucomicrobiota* is low [40]. Alteration in gut microbial composition isrelative togut-brain axis which influence progression of various neurodegenerative diseases. Research conducted a study on the fecal samples of 97 individuals observed lower abundance of *Firmicutes* and higher abundance of *Proteobacteria*, *Gammoproteobacteria*, and *Emterobacteria* in the samples of Alzheimer's patients [20]. Another study reported the increase abundance of *Escherichia/Shigella*and decrease abundance of *E. rectale* in the Alzheimer's patients. Several studies have identified gut microbiota-based biomarker for Alzheimer's disease, however possibility of treating or modifying progression of Alzheimer's disease with microbiome-mediated therapeutics need to be explored more.

It was reported by Braak that gastrointestinal tract is the site where aggregation of α-syn takes place which lead to the initiation of neuroinflammation and dopamine loss in Parkinson's disease [9]. In 15 case studies, it was observed that *Prevotellaceae*, *Lachnospiraceae*, and *Faecalibacterium* were decreased and *Ruminococcaceae*, *Bifidobacteriaceae*, *Christensenellaceae*, and *Verrucomicrobiaceae* were increased in the patients of Parkinson's disease as compared to the healthy individuals [34].

4 Trends of Clinical Genomics Approaches

Tradition clinical genomics includes the Sanger sequencing method which uses chain termination method to sequence the entire genome. To complete the first draft of human genome project took ~13 years [11]. However, further advancement in sequencing technology leads to development of Next Generation Sequencing, which can sequence the complete human genome in a single day. Massively parallel sequencing or deep sequencing has made omics study more useful in the disease analysis and management [5]. This chapter is mainly focusing on two types of sequencing:

4.1 Short-Read Sequencing

Short-read sequencing is used in whole genome sequencing, whole transcriptome sequencing, metagenome sequencing, and whole exome sequencing for gene expression profiling, population genetics, and variant detection. Pyrosequencing, sequencing by synthesis and semiconductor technology are used for short-read sequencing by Roche 454, Illumina and ion torrent respectively.

4.1.1 Pyrosequencing

Chain of enzymatic reactions in pyrosequencing starts with the release of pyrophosphate with the addition of nucleotide by polymerase. Next step begins with the conversion of pyrophosphate to ATP in the presence of ATP sulfurylase followed by transformation of ATP to AMP and luciferin to oxyluciferin in the presence of luciferase. Releasedpyrophosphate can be detected by the emission of light and is the basis of pyrosequencing [28].

4.1.2 Sequencing by Synthesis

Illumina short-read sequencing employs sequencing by synthesis approach. Currently it is the most used sequencing technique due to its high-throughput performance lead by Illumina and known as second next generation sequencing [35].

4.1.3 Semiconductor Technology

Semiconductor technology used by Ion Torrent is also sequencing by synthesis approach. Principle of this method is based on the detection of hydrogen ions during incorporation of nucleotides in the template stand [30].

4.2 Long-Read Sequencing

The contemporary technique to generate long read sequence is called as third next generation sequencing. Long-read sequencing is the best method for determining the sequence of complex DNA sections, such as repeats, while having a larger error in base calling. Long-read sequencing is used for structural variant detection, whole genome sequencing of complex genomes, and sequencing of very repetitive genomes. Oxford Nanopore sequences long DNA or RNA fragments by monitoring the changes to an electrical current when nucleic acids are passed through a protein nanopore [24].

5 Artificial Intelligence (AI) and Machine Learning (ML)

Artificial intelligence is the ability of computer system in mimicking human intelligence to solve problems [33]. ML is a branch of AI which consists of algorithms targeted towards recognizing patterns and extracting noteworthy features from large datasets. After these patterns are identified and learned, ML algorithm can be used to classify and predict results. ML can be used in the diagnosis, prognosis, disease management, and trackingof neurodegenerative diseases. Machine learning approach follows several steps for disease prediction as shown in Fig. 1.

AI and ML for Neurodegenerative Diseases

Electronic medical records and medical images of the patients of neurodegenerative diseases can be analysed using AI and ML for early prediction and analysis of disease. Several types of medicals images (MRI, SPECT, and PET) on neurodegenerative diseases can be analysed using deep learning approach for diagnosis purpose.

- MRI: Clear images of human central nervous system using a large magnet and radio waves. Changes in human brain can be monitored in case of neurodegenerative diseases through repeated scans. Progression and detection of diseases can be analysed by MRI [2, 15]. MRI processing was performed for early detection of Alzheimer's disease [26] using AI approach.
- SPECT: SPECT is an imaging technique which can analyse different organs of the body using gamma rays and can create 3D images. SPECT image was analysed for early detection of Parkinson's disease using Artificial Neural Network [29].

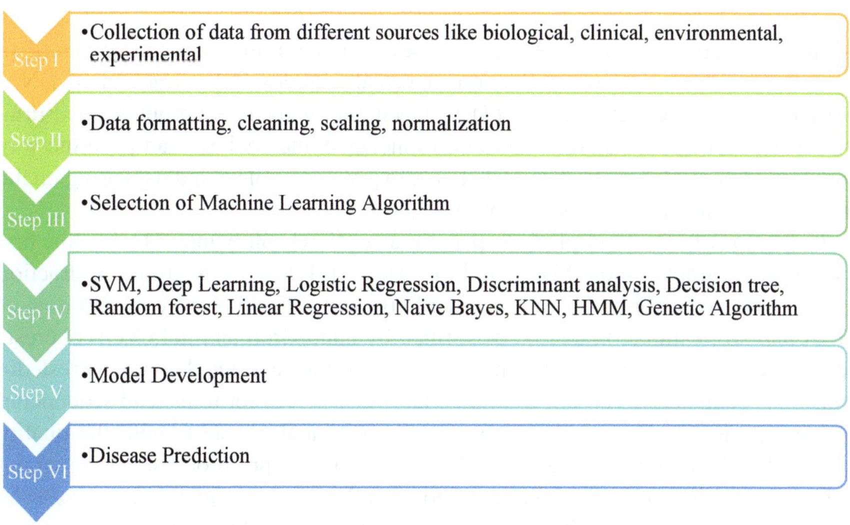

Fig. 1 A schematic representation of the machine learning workflow

Table 1 Different ML algorithms uses in the prediction and classification of Parkinson's disease

ML algorithms	Contributions	Neurodegenerative disease	References
SVM	Diagnosis and classification	Parkinson's Disease	[14]
Random forest	Detection and classification of disease	Parkinson's Disease	[1, 6]
Logistic regression	Classification of disease	Parkinson's Disease	[19]
Deep learning	Prediction and diagnosis of disease	Parkinson's Disease	[32]
Naïve Bayes	Predictive model	Parkinson's Disease	[7]
HMM	Classification of disease	Parkinson's Disease	[18]
KNN	Disease prediction	Parkinson's Disease	[4]

- PET: Generates molecular images which can be used to explore the human neurodegenerative disorders. PET molecular images in Alzheimer's disease is based on the metabolism of glucose in brain. Metabolism of glucose decreases in Alzheimer's disease patients decreased as compared to healthy brain [23].

Table 1 depicts the application of different ML approaches for Parkinson disease.

6 AI and Structure-Based Drug Discovery Approaches in Human Gut Microbiome to Combat Neurodegenerative Disease

Correlation between neurodegenerative diseases and gut microbes can be identified by following the steps: (1) collection of faecal samples, (2) extraction of DNA, (3) metagenome sequencing and (4) metagenome analysis. Computer-aided drug discovery approach, and AI in addition to metagenome analysis can pave the way for development of therapeutics as well as can give a complete understanding on the diseases mechanism and progression (Fig. 2).

Collection of faecal sample from patients as well as healthy individuals is the first step. Faecal samples should be stored in −80 °C till they are analysed. Extraction of DNA can be performed by any standard protocol. Checking the concentration of DNA and size estimation can be performed by nanopdrop and gel electrophoresis respectively. Library preparation and sequencing is the next step. People interestedin short-read sequencing can opt Illumina platform whereas for long-read sequencing Nanopore can be selected. First step in sequence analysis starts with the quality check. If poor quality reads are found in the sequence, pre-processing is essential before any further analysis. Adapter removal and pre-processing are the steps to be followed afterwards. Microbiome sequence assembly is further constructed to identify the microbial (alpha diversity and beta-diversity), taxonomic, and functional

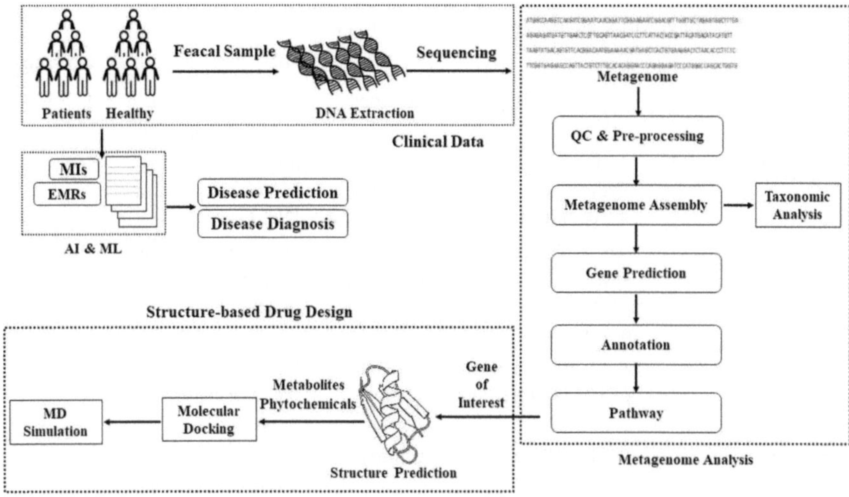

Fig. 2 Pictorial representation of the integrative approach of clinical genomics, structure-based drug design and AI in analysing neurodegenerative diseases

diversities. Gene prediction of the highly abundant phyla can be followed by functional annotation and pathway analysis. Predicted genes of the high abundant and low abundant microbes can further analysed to get insight into the gene ontologies and pathway association. Theanalysis can lead to the identification of some of the important genes which can be targeted to develop therapeutics using structure-based drug design approach. Some of the AI-based tools used in drug discovery approach is presented in Table 2.

Comparative analysis of the gut microbiome in healthy and neurodegenerative disease samples can get insight into the high and low abundant microbes, which can lead to the development of microbiome-based therapeutics. Different probiotics can be used for improving the good microbes in human gut which may alter the gut-brain axis and manage/treat the progression of disease.

Table 2 List of some AI-based tools use in drug discovery

Tools	Details	URL	References
AlphaFold	Protein 3D structure predictions	https://deepmind.com/blog/alphafold	[17]
DeepNeuralNetQSAR	A computationally driven Python-based system for detecting the chemical activity of substances	https://github.com/Merck/DeepNeuralNet-QSAR	[10]
DeepChem	An MLP model that employs an AI system built on Python to identify potential candidates for drug development	https://github.com/deepchem/deepchem	[38]
DeepTox	Software that estimates the toxicity of 12,000 different medications	http://www.bioinf.jku.at/research/DeepTox	[25]
PotentialNet	Predicts ligand binding affinity using NNs	https://pubs.acs.org/doi/full/https://doi.org/10.1021/acscentsci.8b00507	[27]
Hit Dexter	Utilising machine learning to anticipate compounds that may respond to biological tests	http://hitdexter2.zbh.uni-hamburg.de/	[36]
DeltaVina	Rescoring drug-ligand binding affinity using a scoring function	https://github.com/chengwang88/deltavina	[37]
Chemputer	Aids in the standardised reporting of chemical synthesis procedures	https://zenodo.org/record/1481731	[13]

References

1. Açıcı, K., Erdaş, Ç. B., Aşuroğlu, T., Toprak, M. K., Erdem, H., & Oğul, H. (2017). A random forest method to detect Parkinson's disease via gait analysis. In G. Boracchi, L. Iliadis, C. Jayne, & A. Likas (Eds.), *Engineering Applications of Neural Networks* (Vol. 744, pp. 609–619). Springer International Publishing. https://doi.org/10.1007/978-3-319-65172-9_51.
2. Agosta, F., Galantucci, S., & Filippi, M. (2017). Advanced magnetic resonance imaging of neurodegenerative diseases. *Neurological Sciences, 38*(1), 41–51. https://doi.org/10.1007/s10072-016-2764-x
3. Bäckhed, F., Ley, R. E., Sonnenburg, J. L., Peterson, D. A., & Gordon, J. I. (2005). Host-Bacterial Mutualism in the human intestine. *Science, 307*(5717), 1915–1920. https://doi.org/10.1126/science.1104816
4. Bandisode, M. I., Bhanushali, M. R., Singh, M. V., Singh, M. V., & Deshmukh, M. A. (2019). *Prediction of Parkinson Disease Using Knn Algorithm, 6*(4).
5. Behjati, S., & Tarpey, P. S. (2013). What is next generation sequencing? *Archives of Disease in Childhood—Education & Practice Edition, 98*(6), 236–238. https://doi.org/10.1136/archdischild-2013-304340
6. Bharath, E., & Rajagopalana, T. (2023). Parkinson's disease classification using random forest kerb feature selection. *Intelligent Automation & Soft Computing, 36*(2), 1417–1433. https://doi.org/10.32604/iasc.2023.032102
7. Bhatia, D. A., & Sulekh, R. (2017). *Predictive model for Parkinson's disease through Naïve Bayes Classification, 9*(1).

8. Braak, H., & Braak, E. (1991). Neuropathological stageing of Alzheimer-related changes. *Acta Neuropathologica, 82*(4), 239–259. https://doi.org/10.1007/BF00308809
9. Braak, H., R. B, U., Gai, W. P., & Del Tredici, K. (2003). Idiopathic Parkinson's disease: Possible routes by which vulnerable neuronal types may be subject to neuroinvasion by an unknown pathogen. *Journal of Neural Transmission, 110*(5), 517–536.https://doi.org/10.1007/s00702-002-0808-2.
10. Chan, H. C. S., Shan, H., Dahoun, T., Vogel, H., & Yuan, S. (2019). Advancing drug discovery via artificial intelligence. *Trends in Pharmacological Sciences, 40*(8), 592–604. https://doi.org/10.1016/j.tips.2019.06.004
11. Collins, F. S., & Fink, L. (1995). *The human genome project, 19*(3).
12. Erkkinen, M. G., Kim, M.-O., & Geschwind, M. D. (2018). Clinical neurology and epidemiology of the major neurodegenerative diseases. *Cold Spring Harbor Perspectives in Biology, 10*(4), a033118. https://doi.org/10.1101/cshperspect.a033118
13. Gromski, P. S., Granda, J. M., & Cronin, L. (2020). Universal chemical synthesis and discovery with 'The Chemputer.' *Trends in Chemistry, 2*(1), 4–12. https://doi.org/10.1016/j.trechm.2019.07.004
14. Haller, S., Badoud, S., Nguyen, D., Garibotto, V., Lovblad, K. O., & Burkhard, P. R. (2012). Individual detection of patients with parkinson disease using support vector machine analysis of diffusion tensor imaging data: Initial results. *American Journal of Neuroradiology, 33*(11), 2123–2128. https://doi.org/10.3174/ajnr.A3126
15. Hauser, R. A., & Olanow, C. W. (1994). Magnetic resonance imaging of neurodegenerative diseases. *Journal of Neuroimaging, 4*(3), 146–158. https://doi.org/10.1111/jon199443146
16. Hou, Y., Dan, X., Babbar, M., Wei, Y., Hasselbalch, S. G., Croteau, D. L., & Bohr, V. A. (2019). Ageing as a risk factor for neurodegenerative disease. *Nature Reviews Neurology, 15*(10), 565–581. https://doi.org/10.1038/s41582-019-0244-7
17. Jumper, J., Evans, R., Pritzel, A., Green, T., Figurnov, M., Ronneberger, O., Tunyasuvunakool, K., Bates, R., Žídek, A., Potapenko, A., Bridgland, A., Meyer, C., Kohl, S. A. A., Ballard, A. J., Cowie, A., Romera-Paredes, B., Nikolov, S., Jain, R., Adler, J., … Hassabis, D. (2021). Highly accurate protein structure prediction with AlphaFold. *Nature, 596*(7873), 583–589.https://doi.org/10.1038/s41586-021-03819-2
18. Khorasani, A., & Daliri, M. R. (2014). HMM for classification of Parkinson's disease based on the raw gait data. *Journal of Medical Systems, 38*(12), 147. https://doi.org/10.1007/s10916-014-0147-5
19. Kim, J.-W., Kwon, Y., Yun, J.-S., Heo, J.-H., Eom, G.-M., Tack, G.-R., Lim, T.-H., & Koh, S.-B. (2015). Regression models for the quantification of Parkinsonian bradykinesia. *Bio-Medical Materials and Engineering, 26*(s1), S2249–S2258. https://doi.org/10.3233/BME-151531
20. Liu, P., Wu, L., Peng, G., Han, Y., Tang, R., Ge, J., Zhang, L., Jia, L., Yue, S., Zhou, K., Li, L., Luo, B., & Wang, B. (2019). Altered microbiomes distinguish Alzheimer's disease from amnestic mild cognitive impairment and health in a Chinese cohort. *Brain, Behavior, and Immunity, 80*, 633–643. https://doi.org/10.1016/j.bbi.2019.05.008
21. Lloyd-Price, J., Abu-Ali, G., & Huttenhower, C. (2016). The healthy human microbiome. *Genome Medicine, 8*(1), 51. https://doi.org/10.1186/s13073-016-0307-y
22. Long, J. M., & Holtzman, D. M. (2019). Alzheimer disease: An update on pathobiology and treatment strategies. *Cell, 179*(2), 312–339. https://doi.org/10.1016/j.cell.2019.09.001
23. Lu, F.-M., & Yuan, Z. (2015). PET/SPECT molecular imaging in clinical neuroscience: Recent advances in the investigation of CNS diseases. *Quantitative Imaging in Medicine and Surgery, 5*(3).
24. Mantere, T., Kersten, S., & Hoischen, A. (2019). Long-read sequencing emerging in medical genetics. *Frontiers in Genetics, 10*, 426. https://doi.org/10.3389/fgene.2019.00426
25. Mayr, A., Klambauer, G., Unterthiner, T., & Hochreiter, S. (2016). DeepTox: Toxicity prediction using deep learning. *Frontiers in Environmental Science, 3.* https://doi.org/10.3389/fenvs.2015.00080

26. Pan, D., Zeng, A., Jia, L., Huang, Y., Frizzell, T., & Song, X. (2020). Early Detection of Alzheimer's disease using magnetic resonance imaging: A novel approach combining convolutional neural networks and ensemble learning. *Frontiers in Neuroscience, 14*, 259. https://doi.org/10.3389/fnins.2020.00259
27. Pereira, J. C., Caffarena, E. R., & Dos Santos, C. N. (2016). Boosting docking-based virtual screening with deep learning. *Journal of Chemical Information and Modeling, 56*(12), 2495–2506. https://doi.org/10.1021/acs.jcim.6b00355
28. Ronaghi, M. (n.d.). *Pyrosequencing sheds light on DNA sequencing.*
29. Rumman, M., Tasneem, A. N., Farzana, S., Pavel, M. I., & Alam, Md. A. (2018). Early detection of Parkinson's disease using image processing and artificial neural network. *2018 Joint 7th International Conference on Informatics, Electronics & Vision (ICIEV) and 2018 2nd International Conference on Imaging, Vision & Pattern Recognition (IcIVPR)*, 256–261. https://doi.org/10.1109/ICIEV.2018.8641081
30. Salipante, S. J., Kawashima, T., Rosenthal, C., Hoogestraat, D. R., Cummings, L. A., Sengupta, D. J., Harkins, T. T., Cookson, B. T., & Hoffman, N. G. (2014). Performance comparison of Illumina and Ion torrent next-generation sequencing platforms for 16S rRNA-based bacterial community profiling. *Applied and Environmental Microbiology, 80*(24), 7583–7591. https://doi.org/10.1128/AEM.02206-14
31. Sender, R., Fuchs, S., & Milo, R. (2016). Revised estimates for the number of human and bacteria cells in the body. *PLOS Biology, 14*(8), e1002533. https://doi.org/10.1371/journal.pbio.1002533
32. Shahid, A. H., & Singh, M. P. (2020). A deep learning approach for prediction of Parkinson's disease progression. *Biomedical Engineering Letters, 10*(2), 227–239. https://doi.org/10.1007/s13534-020-00156-7
33. Sheikh, H., Prins, C., & Schrijvers, E. (2023). *Mission AI: The new system technology*. Springer International Publishing.https://doi.org/10.1007/978-3-031-21448-6
34. Shen, T., Yue, Y., He, T., Huang, C., Qu, B., Lv, W., & Lai, H.-Y. (2021). The Association between the gut microbiota and Parkinson's disease, a meta-analysis. *Frontiers in Aging Neuroscience, 13*, 636545. https://doi.org/10.3389/fnagi.2021.636545
35. Simon, S. A., Zhai, J., Nandety, R. S., McCormick, K. P., Zeng, J., Mejia, D., & Meyers, B. C. (2009). Short-read sequencing technologies for transcriptional analyses. *Annual Review of Plant Biology, 60*(1), 305–333. https://doi.org/10.1146/annurev.arplant.043008.092032
36. Stork, C., Chen, Y., Šícho, M., & Kirchmair, J. (2019). Hit Dexter 2.0: Machine-learning models for the prediction of frequent hitters. *Journal of Chemical Information and Modeling, 59*(3), 1030–1043. https://doi.org/10.1021/acs.jcim.8b00677
37. Wang, C., & Zhang, Y. (2017). Improving scoring-docking-screening powers of protein-ligand scoring functions using random forest. *Journal of Computational Chemistry, 38*(3), 169–177. https://doi.org/10.1002/jcc.24667
38. Zhu, H. (2020). Big data and artificial intelligence modeling for drug discovery. *Annual Review of Pharmacology and Toxicology, 60*(1), 573–589. https://doi.org/10.1146/annurev-pharmtox-010919-023324
39. Zhu, M., Liu, X., Ye, Y., Yan, X., Cheng, Y., Zhao, L., Chen, F., & Ling, Z. (2022). Gut microbiota: A novel therapeutic target for Parkinson's disease. *Frontiers in Immunology, 13*, 937555. https://doi.org/10.3389/fimmu.2022.937555
40. Zoetendal, E. G., Akkermans, A. D. L., & De Vos, W. M. (1998). Temperature gradient gel electrophoresis analysis of 16S rRNA from human Fecal samples reveals stable and host-specific communities of active Bacteria. *Applied and Environmental Microbiology, 64*(10), 3854–3859. https://doi.org/10.1128/AEM.64.10.3854-3859.1998

Amyotrophic Lateral Sclerosis (ALS) Monitoring Using Explainable AI

Loveleen Gaur and Devanshi Gaur

Abstract Amyotrophic Lateral Sclerosis (ALS), often referred to as Lou Gehrig's disease, is a rare and debilitating neurodegenerative disorder that affects motor neurons in the brain and spinal cord. It leads to the progressive degeneration of these neurons, resulting in muscle weakness, loss of motor function, and, eventually, paralysis. Monitoring the progression of ALS is critical for timely interventions and personalized care. In recent years, eXplainable Artificial Intelligence (XAI) has emerged as a powerful tool in the field of ALS monitoring and management. ALS is a highly heterogeneous disease, meaning it manifests differently in each patient. Some individuals may experience rapid progression, while others have a slower course. Monitoring this variability and tailoring interventions accordingly is where XAI can make a substantial impact.

Keywords Explainable Artificial Intelligence · Neurodegenerative Diseases · Advancements in Neuroimaging · Amyotrophic Lateral Sclerosis

1 Introduction

In the vast landscape of medicine and healthcare, there are moments when the potential of cutting-edge technology confronts the harsh realities posed by relentless and devastating diseases. Amyotrophic Lateral Sclerosis (ALS) represents one such challenge, serving as a poignant reminder of the profound intricacies within the human body and the pressing need for innovative solutions to address its relentless progression.

ALS, also known as Lou Gehrig's disease, is a cruel adversary that operates silently, gradually and irreversibly eroding a person's ability to perform even the

L. Gaur (✉)
Taylor's University, Subang Jaya, Malaysia
e-mail: gaurloveleen@yahoo.com

D. Gaur
Florida International University, Miami, USA
e-mail: dgaur002@fiu.edu

© The Author(s), under exclusive license to Springer Nature Switzerland AG 2024

L. Gaur et al. (eds.), *AI and Neuro-Degenerative Diseases*, Studies in Computational Intelligence 1131, https://doi.org/10.1007/978-3-031-53148-4_5

most basic tasks. It begins with subtle muscle weakness, often going unnoticed until it manifests in more severe symptoms like difficulty in speaking, swallowing, or moving. Ultimately, ALS robs individuals of their independence and, eventually, their lives.

As the medical community battles this formidable foe, a new and promising ally emerges from the realm of Artificial Intelligence (AI)—eXplainable AI (XAI). XAI, with its unique ability to provide clear and interpretable insights into complex data, offers a ray of hope in the quest to monitor, understand, and ultimately combat this debilitating condition [1–5].

However, the introduction of XAI into the field of ALS monitoring is not merely a scientific development but a profound intersection of technology and humanity. It prompts us to contemplate the implications and consequences of relying on machines to navigate the delicate and deeply personal journey of a patient grappling with a neurodegenerative disease.

In this exploration, we embark on a thought-provoking journey into the world of Amyotrophic Lateral Sclerosis monitoring using XAI. It's a journey that raises profound questions about the evolving relationship between technology and the human experience in the context of healthcare. We will discover how XAI not only offers hope for improved ALS care but also challenges our understanding of ethics, empathy, and the fundamental aspects of what it means to be human when technology enters the equation.

2 Role of XAI in ALS Monitoring

The role of eXplainable Artificial Intelligence (XAI) in ALS (Amyotrophic Lateral Sclerosis) monitoring is multifaceted and holds significant potential in improving patient care, disease management, and research. Here are several key aspects of how XAI can contribute to ALS monitoring:

1. **Data Integration and Analysis**: One of the key strengths of XAI is its ability to integrate and analyze diverse data sources [6]. In the context of ALS monitoring, this includes:

    - *Clinical Records*: XAI can process historical clinical data, including motor function assessments, electromyography (EMG) results, and patient-reported outcomes. By analyzing this information, XAI can identify trends and patterns indicative of disease progression.
    - *Genetic Information*: Genetic factors play a role in ALS susceptibility and progression. XAI can analyze genetic data to identify relevant genetic markers and their influence on disease course.
    - *Wearable Devices*: Wearable sensors can continuously monitor patients' motor function, speech patterns, and other vital signs. XAI algorithms can process this real-time data and provide insights into daily fluctuations in a patient's condition.

- *Multi-Source Data Integration*: ALS monitoring often requires the integration of various data sources, including clinical records, genetic information, electromyography (EMG) results, and wearable device data [7]. XAI excels in processing and integrating these diverse data types to provide a comprehensive view of the patient's condition.
- *Pattern Recognition*: XAI can identify subtle patterns and trends within patient data, which can be challenging for human observers to detect. This includes changes in motor function, muscle strength, and respiratory capacity, all of which are critical indicators of ALS progression[8–10].

2. **Disease Progression Prediction**: XAI can develop predictive models that estimate the likely trajectory of ALS progression for individual patients. By considering various factors, such as changes in motor function, muscle strength, and respiratory capacity, these models can provide valuable information to clinicians. This allows for the early adjustment of treatment plans and interventions as needed.

   - *Predictive Models*: XAI can develop predictive models that estimate the likely trajectory of ALS progression for individual patients. By considering historical data and a range of relevant factors, such as clinical assessments and genetic profiles, these models can provide valuable insights into how the disease is expected to evolve over time [11–15].
   - *Early Detection*: XAI can detect early signs of disease progression, allowing healthcare providers to intervene proactively. For instance, it can predict when a patient may require respiratory support or changes in medication regimens.

3. **Treatment Response Assessment**: ALS patients often undergo various treatments and therapies aimed at managing symptoms and slowing disease progression. XAI can assess the effectiveness of these treatments by analyzing patient data over time. It can help identify which interventions yield the most significant benefits, allowing for personalized treatment plans.

   - *Personalized Treatment Plans*: ALS patients often undergo various treatments and therapies, but responses can vary widely among individuals. XAI can assess the effectiveness of these treatments by analyzing patient data over time. It helps identify which interventions are most beneficial for specific patients, enabling personalized treatment plans.

4. **Continuous Monitoring and Alerts**:

   - *Real-time Data Analysis*: Wearable devices equipped with sensors can collect real-time data on ALS patients, monitoring motor function, speech patterns, and other vital signs. XAI algorithms can continuously analyze this data, providing timely alerts to healthcare providers when it detects concerning changes or complications.

- *Respiratory Support Alerts*: XAI can predict when a patient's respiratory function may decline, enabling the timely initiation of non-invasive or invasive ventilation, a crucial aspect of ALS care.

5. **Symptom Management**:

- *Speech and Swallowing*: XAI can monitor changes in speech patterns and swallowing abilities, common challenges in ALS. It can offer recommendations for adaptive technologies or therapeutic strategies to maintain communication and adequate nutrition [16, 17].

6. **Patient-Specific Recommendations**:

- *Personalized Care Plans*: XAI generates personalized recommendations for ALS patients based on their unique data profiles. These recommendations may include specific exercises, dietary guidelines, or assistive devices tailored to each patient's needs, improving their quality of life and independence.

7. **Data Visualization and Interpretability**:

- *Transparent Insights*: XAI provides interpretable visualizations of patient data, allowing both healthcare providers and patients to better understand disease progression and the impact of various factors. Transparent insights facilitate shared decision-making and patient engagement in their care.

8. **Clinical Trial Design**:

- *Efficient Trials*: XAI can assist in designing more efficient and effective clinical trials for potential ALS treatments by identifying suitable patient cohorts and optimizing trial protocols. This can accelerate the development of new therapies.

9. **Ethical Considerations**:

- *Data Privacy and Informed Consent*: Ensuring ethical considerations, such as data privacy and informed consent, is paramount in ALS monitoring. XAI can help uphold these principles by providing transparent and accountable data processing and analysis.

eXplainable Artificial Intelligence (XAI) offers significant advantages in the monitoring and management of Amyotrophic Lateral Sclerosis (ALS) [18–21]. By integrating and analyzing diverse data sources, predicting disease progression, assessing treatment responses, and offering personalized recommendations, XAI empowers healthcare providers to deliver more effective, patient-centered care. As ALS is a complex and variable disease, XAI's ability to provide transparent insights into the disease's progression is invaluable for tailoring interventions and improving patients' quality of life. Ongoing research and collaborations between AI experts and ALS clinicians will likely continue to advance the role of XAI in ALS monitoring and care.

3 Challenges in Implementing XAI in ALS Monitoring

- *Data Heterogeneity*: ALS monitoring involves integrating diverse data sources, including clinical records, genetic data, and real-time sensor data from wearable devices. Ensuring the seamless integration and preprocessing of these heterogeneous data sets can be challenging.
- *Data Volume and Scalability*: As data is continuously generated in real-time, managing and processing large volumes of data becomes a significant challenge. XAI algorithms need to be scalable to handle the growing data streams effectively.
- *Interpretable Models*: While XAI promotes model interpretability, achieving the right balance between model complexity and interpretability can be difficult. Complex models may offer higher accuracy but may be less interpretable, making it challenging to gain insights from them.
- *Ethical and Privacy Concerns*: ALS monitoring often involves sensitive patient data. Ensuring data privacy, informed consent, and ethical data usage is crucial. Balancing the need for data access with patient privacy protection is an ongoing challenge.
- *Lack of Standardization*: There is a lack of standardized data collection and monitoring protocols in ALS care. This heterogeneity can hinder the development and deployment of XAI models across different healthcare settings.
- *Patient Variability*: ALS progression varies significantly among patients. Developing personalized XAI models that can adapt to individual patient profiles is a complex task.
- *Clinical Validation*: XAI models need rigorous clinical validation to ensure their reliability and effectiveness in real-world ALS monitoring scenarios. This requires collaboration between AI researchers and healthcare professionals [22–24].

4 Future Directions for Research and Development

- *Improved Data Integration*: Future research can focus on developing more efficient methods for integrating heterogeneous data sources in ALS monitoring. This may involve creating standardized data formats and interoperable healthcare systems.
- *Scalable XAI Algorithms*: The development of XAI algorithms that can scale to handle large volumes of data efficiently is crucial. Research in this area can lead to more robust and scalable models.
- *Hybrid Models*: Future XAI models can explore hybrid approaches that combine the interpretability of rule-based models with the predictive power of deep learning, striking a balance between accuracy and transparency.
- *Ethical Frameworks*: Researchers should continue to work on ethical frameworks for AI and XAI in healthcare. These frameworks should address issues of data privacy, consent, and fairness in AI-driven ALS monitoring.

- *Personalized Monitoring*: Advancements in AI and XAI can lead to more personalized ALS monitoring, where models adapt to the unique characteristics and needs of each patient, enhancing the quality of care.
- *Clinical Trials Optimization*: XAI can be further utilized to optimize clinical trial design, speeding up the development of new ALS treatments. Research can focus on developing AI-driven trial design tools.
- *Patient-Centric Approaches*: Future research should prioritize patient-centric approaches, involving ALS patients in the design and development of monitoring systems to ensure they meet real-world needs and are user-friendly.
- *Data Sharing and Collaboration*: Encouraging collaboration between institutions and researchers to share data and insights can accelerate the development and validation of XAI models for ALS monitoring.
- *Regulatory Frameworks*: The development of regulatory frameworks specific to AI and XAI in healthcare can provide guidance on ethical, legal, and safety standards for ALS monitoring systems.
- *Longitudinal Studies*: Conducting long-term studies that track ALS patients over extended periods can provide valuable data for training and validating XAI models, improving their accuracy and reliability.

While there are challenges in implementing XAI in ALS monitoring, ongoing research and development efforts hold the promise of addressing these challenges and advancing the field. Future directions should focus on improving data integration, model scalability, ethics, and personalization while fostering collaboration and regulatory frameworks to ensure the responsible and effective use of XAI in ALS care [25–27].

5 Conclusion

XAI holds the potential to significantly enhance ALS care by integrating, analyzing, and interpreting diverse patient data sources, including clinical records, genetics, and real-time sensor data from wearables. XAI models can predict ALS progression, treatment responses, and early signs of complications. This predictive power aids in personalized treatment planning and timely interventions. The wearable devices equipped with sensors, when coupled with XAI, offer continuous real-time monitoring. XAI analyzes this data, providing alerts for potential issues. XAI provides interpretable insights into complex patient data, allowing both healthcare providers and patients to understand disease progression and the impact of various factors clearly. XAI enables personalized care plans tailored to individual patient profiles, improving the patient's quality of life and independence. XAI can optimize clinical trial design, potentially accelerating the development of new ALS treatments.

References

1. Antoniadi, A. M., Galvin, M., Heverin, M., et al. (2021). Prediction of caregiver quality of life in amyotrophic lateral sclerosis using explainable machine learning. *Science and Reports, 11*, 12237. https://doi.org/10.1038/s41598-021-91632-2
2. Bhandari, M., Neupane, A., Mallik, S., Gaur, L., & Qin, H. (2023). Auguring fake face images using dual input convolution neural network. *Journal of Imaging, 9*(1), 3. https://doi.org/10.3390/jimaging9010003
3. Gaur, L., & Sahoo, B. M. (2022). Introduction to explainable AI and intelligent transportation. In *Explainable artificial intelligence for intelligent transportation systems*. Springer. https://doi.org/10.1007/978-3-031-09644-0_1
4. Antoniadi, A. M., Galvin, M., Heverin, M., Wei, L., Hardiman, O., & Mooney, C. (2022). A clinical decision support system for the prediction of quality of life in ALS. *Journal of Personalized Medicine, 12*(3), 435. https://doi.org/10.3390/jpm12030435.PMID:35330435;PMCID:PMC8955774
5. Papaiz, F., Dourado, M. E. T., Jr., Valentim, R. A. M., Morais, A. H. F., & Arrais, J. P. (2022). Machine learning solutions applied to amyotrophic lateral sclerosis prognosis: A review. *Frontiers in Computer Science, 4*, 869140. https://doi.org/10.3389/fcomp.2022.869140
6. Di Martino, F., & Delmastro, F. (2023). Explainable AI for clinical and remote health applications: A survey on tabular and time series data. *Artificial Intelligence Review, 56*, 5261–5315. https://doi.org/10.1007/s10462-022-10304-3
7. Shortliffe, E. H., & Buchanan, B.G.: A model of inexact reasoning in medicine. *Mathematical Biosciences, 23*, 351–379 (1975). https://doi.org/10.1016/0025-5564(75)90047-4
8. Lindsay, R. K., Buchanan, B. G., Feigenbaum, E. A., Lederberg, J. (1993). DENDRAL: A case study of the first expert system for scientific hypothesis formation. *Artificial Intelligence, 61*, 209–261. https://doi.org/10.1016/0004-3702(93)90068-M
9. Miller, R. A., Pople, H. E. J., & Myers, J. D. (1982). Internist-1, an experimental computer-based diagnostic consultant for general internal medicine. *New England Journal of Medicine, 307*, 468–476. https://doi.org/10.1056/NEJM198208193070803
10. de Dombal, F. T., Leaper, D. J., Staniland, J. R., McCann, A. P., & Horrocks, J. C. (1972). Computer-aided diagnosis of acute abdominal pain. *British Medical Journal, 2*, 9–13. https://doi.org/10.1136/bmj.2.5804.9
11. Ghose, P., Alavi, M., Tabassum, M., Ashraf Uddin, M., Biswas, M., Mahbub, K., Gaur, L., Mallik, S., & Zhao, Z. (2022). Detecting COVID-19 infection status from chest X-ray and CT scan via single transfer learning-driven approach. *Frontiers in Genetics, 13*, 980338. https://doi.org/10.3389/fgene.2022.980338
12. Gaur, L., Bhandari, M., Razdan, T., Mallik, S., & Zhao, Z. (2022). Explanation-driven deep learning model for prediction of brain tumour status using MRI image data. *Frontiers in Genetics, 13*, 822666. https://doi.org/10.3389/fgene.2022.822666
13. De Fauw, J., Ledsam, J. R., Romera-Paredes, B., Nikolov, S., Tomasev, N., Blackwell, S., Askham, H., Glorot, X., O'Donoghue, B., Visentin, D., van den Driessche, G., Lakshminarayanan, B., Meyer, C., Mackinder, F., Bouton, S., Ayoub, K., Chopra, R., King, D., Karthikesalingam, A., … Ronneberger, O. (2018). Clinically applicable deep learning for diagnosis and referral in retinal disease. *Nature Medicine, 24*, 1342–1350. https://doi.org/10.1038/s41591-018-0107-6
14. Bhandari, M., Parajuli, P., Chapagain, P., & Gaur, L. (2022). Evaluating performance of Adam optimization by proposing energy index. In K. Santosh, R. Hegadi, & U. Pal (Eds.), *Recent trends in image processing and pattern recognition. RTIP2R 2021. Communications in computer and information science* (vol. 1576). Springer. https://doi.org/10.1007/978-3-031-07005-1_15
15. Raghupathi, W., & Raghupathi, V. (2014). Big data analytics in healthcare: Promise and potential. *Health Information Science and Systems, 2*, 3. https://doi.org/10.1186/2047-2501-2-3

16. Alzubaidi, L., Zhang, J., Humaidi, A. J., Al-Dujaili, A., Duan, Y., Al-Shamma, O., Santamaría, J., Fadhel, M. A., Al-Amidie, M., & Farhan, L. (2021). Review of deep learning: Concepts, CNN architectures, challenges, applications, future directions. *Springer International Publishing*. https://doi.org/10.1186/s40537-021-00444-8
17. Pyrros, A., Rodriguez Fernandez, J., Borstelmann, S. M., Flanders, A., Wenzke, D., Hart, E., Horowitz, J. M., Nikolaidis, P., Willis, M., Chen, A., Cole, P., Siddiqui, N., Muzaffar, M., Muzaffar, N., McVean, J., Menchaca, M., Katsaggelos, A. K., Koyejo, S., & Galanter, W. (2022). Validation of a deep learning, value-based care model to predict mortality and comorbidities from chest radiographs in COVID-19. *PLOS Digital Health, 1*, e0000057. https://doi.org/10.1371/journal.pdig.0000057
18. Wang, L., Li, P., Hou, M., Zhang, X., Cao, X., & Li, H. (2021). Construction of a risk prediction model for Alzheimer's disease in the elderly population. *BMC Neurology, 21*, 271. https://doi.org/10.1186/s12883-021-02276-8
19. Gaur, L., Singh, G., & Agarwal, V. (2021). Leveraging artificial intelligence tools to combat the COVID-19 crisis. In P. K. Singh, G. Veselov, V. Vyatkin, A. Pljonkin, J. M. Dodero, & Y. Kumar (Eds.), *Futuristic trends in network and communication technologies. FTNCT 2020. Communications in computer and information science* (vol. 1395). Springer. https://doi.org/10.1007/978-981-16-1480-4_28
20. Sweeney, L. (2002). K-anonymity: A model for protecting privacy. *International Journal of Uncertainty, Fuzziness and Knowledge-Based Systems, 10*, 557–570. https://doi.org/10.1142/S0218488502001648
21. Saeed, S., Haroon, H. B., Naqvi, M., Jhanjhi, N. Z., Ahmad, M., & Gaur, L. (2022). A systematic mapping study of low-grade tumor of brain cancer and CSF fluid detecting approaches and parameters. In N. Zaman, L. Gaur, & M. Humayun (Eds.), *Approaches and applications of deep learning in virtual medical care* (pp. 236–259). IGI Global. https://doi.org/10.4018/978-1-7998-8929-8.ch010
22. Gaur, L., Bhatia, U., & Bakshi, S. (2022). Cloud driven framework for skin cancer detection using deep CNN. In *2022 2nd international conference on innovative practices in technology and management (ICIPTM)* (pp. 460–464). https://doi.org/10.1109/ICIPTM54933.2022.9754216
23. Ghose, P., Sharmin, S., Gaur, L., & Zhao, Z. (2022). Grid-search integrated optimized support vector machine model for breast cancer detection. In *2022 IEEE international conference on bioinformatics and biomedicine (BIBM)* (pp. 2846–2852). https://doi.org/10.1109/BIBM55620.2022.9995703
24. Gaur, L., Jhanjhi, N. Z., Bakshi, S., & Gupta, P. (2022). Analyzing consequences of artificial intelligence on jobs using topic modeling and keyword extraction. In *2022 2nd international conference on innovative practices in technology and management (ICIPTM)* (pp. 435–440). https://doi.org/10.1109/ICIPTM54933.2022.9754064
25. Antoniadi, A. M. et al. (2021). Prediction of quality of life in people with ALS: On the road towards explainable clinical decision support. *ACM SIGAPP Applied Computing Review, 21*(2), 5–17. https://doi.org/10.1145/3477127.3477128
26. Kormas, P., & Moutzouri, A. (2020). Current psychological approaches in neurodegenerative diseases. In P. Vlamos, I. S. Kotsireas, & I. Tarnanas (Eds.), *Handbook of Computational Neurodegeneration* (pp. 1–29). Springer International Publishing. https://doi.org/10.1007/978-3-319-75479-6_10-1
27. Gaur, L., Bhatia, U., Jhanjhi, N. Z., et al. (2023). Medical image-based detection of COVID-19 using deep convolution neural networks. *Multimedia Systems, 29*, 1729–1738. https://doi.org/10.1007/s00530-021-00794-6

Prevalence of Dementia in India

Sandeep Bhasin and Bhawna Kumar

Abstract Dementia, a complex and debilitating neurodegenerative disorder, poses a significant public health challenge worldwide. This research aims to investigate the prevalence of dementia in India, shedding light on the demographic and regional variations in this rapidly evolving landscape. Utilizing a comprehensive cross-sectional study design, data was collected from diverse urban and rural populations across the country. The study employed standardized research tools to evaluate cognitive function and diagnose dementia cases. Our findings reveal a nuanced picture of dementia prevalence in India, emphasizing the influence of socio-economic factors, lifestyle, and regional disparities. The implications of our research extend beyond epidemiological insights, offering a foundation for targeted interventions, policy development, and healthcare planning to address the growing burden of dementia in the Indian population. This paper contributes to the global discourse on dementia by presenting a detailed analysis of its prevalence in a dynamic and diverse socio-cultural context.

Keywords Dementia · Neurodegenerative disorders · Cognitive impairment · Epidemiology · Public health · India · Prevalence · Demographics · Cross-sectional study · Regional variations

1 Introduction

Dementia is a medical condition that impacts cognitive and social abilities, posing challenges for individuals in performing their everyday tasks. It is a comprehensive term that encompasses various cognitive impairments and neurodegenerative disorders, resulting in functional and behavioural difficulties. These challenges arise from a notable decline in mental capacity that significantly hampers daily life. Memory

S. Bhasin (✉)
InnovoElixir Consulting, New Delhi, India
e-mail: sbhasin@outlook.com

B. Kumar
Australian School of Global Studies, Sydney, Australia

© The Author(s), under exclusive license to Springer Nature Switzerland AG 2024
L. Gaur et al. (eds.), *AI and Neuro-Degenerative Diseases*, Studies in Computational Intelligence 1131, https://doi.org/10.1007/978-3-031-53148-4_6

loss is a prime example of such an issue. While Alzheimer's disease stands as the most prevalent form of dementia, it is just one among several types. The term "dementia" originates from the Latin word "demens," meaning "out of one's mind." Presently, "dementia" ranks among the top 10,000 most frequently used words in the Collins dictionary.

Over 70% of dementia cases worldwide come from the patients of Alzheimer's disease. Alzheimer's, also known as amyloid-β, is an incurable neurodegenerative disorder where a brain slowly destroys memory and thinking skills and, eventually, the ability to carry out some of the easiest tasks [1]. The scientists are yet to understand the cause of Alzheimer's disease [2] although it is generally accepted that genetic factors, Age and lifestyle may add to the development of Alzheimer's in patients [3]. In the United States alone, over 6 million people are estimated to have Alzheimer's disease. Worldwide, this figure crosses over 40 million, with over 20 million from low income nations [4]. It is estimated that close to 8.80 million Indians (7.4% of people above the age of 60 years live with dementia, it is more prevalent in women and in rural India [5]. According to World Health Organization [6], 10 million new cases of dementia are expected to get added every year going forward. This number will almost double every 20 years, reaching 78 million in 2030 and 139 million in 2050 [7]. One in ten individuals aged greater than 65 years has Alzheimer's and its incidence continues to increase with age. In humans, tissues predominantly consisting of postmitotic cells are susceptible to the impacts of the aging process. Various factors such as genomic instability, telomere attrition, epigenetic changes, loss of proteostasis, mitochondrial dysfunction, cellular senescence, disrupted nutrient sensing, stem cell depletion, and altered intercellular communication are closely associated with vulnerability to neurodegenerative diseases [8]. The cost of dementia to the nations globally was around USD 1.3 trillion [6]. Approximately 50% of this cost was attributed to the informal care providers. With limited understanding of the brain structure and its functions, it has become a major challenge for the researchers early diagnosis of disease, but generally accepted risks are age (65 or older), high blood pressure (hypertension), high blood sugar (diabetes), being overweight or obese, smoking and/or drinking too much alcohol, being physically inactive, being socially isolated and depression [9]. The interconnection between physical and mental illnesses, especially in old age, must be understood. Whether it is diabetes, high blood pressure or hypertension, thyroid issues, prostate problems, osteoarthritis or knee pain, a link with mental health conditions is inevitable [10]. Alzheimer's disease among the elderly (including other dementias) increased by close to 150% between 1990 and 2019, with 2.92 million cases in 1990 and 7.24 million cases in 2019 [11]. Cardiovascular risk factors, such as diabetes and hypertension, also have an effect on cerebral vasculature, which in turn, can increase the risk of stroke and dementia [12]. This adds to the issue of multiple diseases leading to dementia in the elderly, thus creating a challenge for the scientists to prioritize either the prevention or the cure of dementia. We have already seen some preventive suggestions being popularised by the scientists such as physical activities, thinking activities, eating healthy etc. However, there is no strong scientific proof of these measures working towards prevention of the neurogenerative diseases, although there's a strong belief on it, none the less. A recent publication in Lancet Public Health supports the forecast that the number will skyrocket (Figs. 1 and 2). The study predicts that by 2050, the number will increase threefold to 152.8 million, with women being disproportionately impacted by the condition [13]. According to the study undertaken by Nichols et al., the occurrence of dementia was more common in women compared to men and rose with age. It doubled approximately every 5 years until the age of 85 in both 2019 and 2050 [13].

2 Aging and Dementia

Aging is an inevitable part of our life. Over the last 100 years, the average human lifespan has increased by approximately 30 years. This demographic shift has resulted in a large population of older citizens. As we age, our knowledge and experience increase, but our cognitive abilities greatly decline. Dementia, a progressive deterioration of cognitive function, is one of the most under-recognized and under-treated chronic conditions in the world today, and India is no different. Close to 90% of dementia patients go undetected and untreated [14]. Improvements in diagnostic methods and treatment protocols have led to an increase in human lifespan. However, dementia often goes undiagnosed, and a definitive treatment for most cases of dementia is still not available [15].

The cognitive response of human body, which is a vital aspect of brain health which includes clarity in thinking and learning, and memory, is maintained by taking care of physical health, eating a healthy, staying socially connected, and engaging in physical exercise. Additionally, the mind and body are kept active through cognitive training. The ability to adapt and develop new abilities throughout our lives is possessed by our brains, although this varies from person to person. Neuroplasticity[1] is known as the ability to reorganize and create new ways to develop cognitive functions. Memory decline with age is not always resulted in by the neurocognitive status of the brain; sometimes it results in preservation or even improvement. This complex relationship largely depends on the specific area of the brain involved [15]. For example, working memory, which is controlled by the prefrontal cortex, tends to be significantly declined with age. In contrast, less reduction in functioning is shown by episodic memory, which is mediated by the hippocampus [16].

Mild cognitive impairment is a condition that often comes before dementia. In this condition, the decline in cognitive abilities, especially memory, is more than what is expected for a person's age. However, it usually does not affect a person's ability to carry out their daily activities independently [17]. In contrast, even in its early stages, dementia is characterized by a clear loss of the ability to function independently. This

[1] Neuroplasticity refers to the brain's capacity to undergo changes and adapt in response to novel experiences. In other words, the brain can reorganize its neural connections and create new pathways to help us learn, remember, and recover from injury. While it was once thought that this ability was limited to childhood, research has shown that the brain can continue to change and adapt throughout our lives.

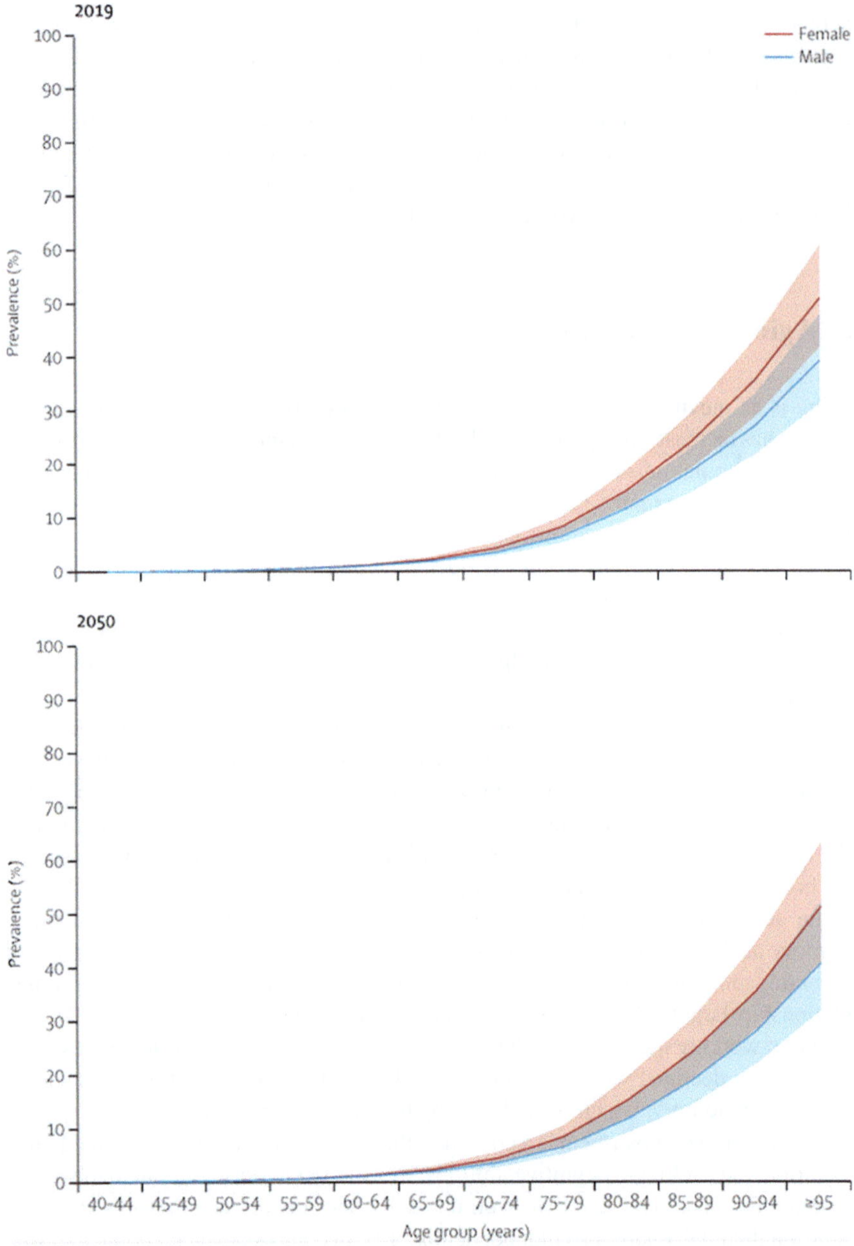

Fig. 1 Global prevalence of dementia (with 95% uncertainty intervals) by age group and sex in 2019 and 2050 [13]

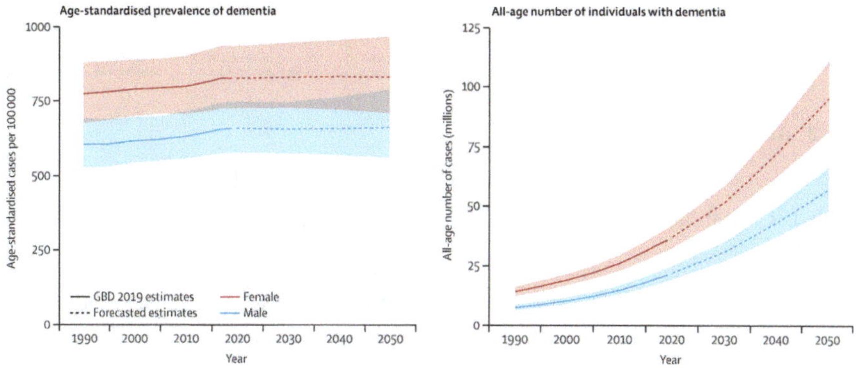

Fig. 2 Estimated trends in the global age-standardised dementia prevalence (**a**) and all-age number of cases (**b**), with 95% uncertainty intervals, 2019–50 [13]

is accompanied by progressive changes in cognitive and behavioural abilities [17]. Doctors classify dementia as 'primary' or 'secondary'. Basis the disease progression, it can also be categorized as 'reversible' or 'irreversible'. In the reversible type, symptoms may be caused by one or more medical conditions that can be treated [15].

3 Understanding Clinical Dementia Rating

The Washington University's Clinical Dementia Rating (CDR) is a globally recognized scale used to determine the incidence and severity of dementia of the Alzheimer's type (DAT). It involves unstructured interviews with both the patient and the family member/attendant to assess cognitive performance in six areas: memory, orientation, judgment and problem solving, community affairs, home and hobbies, and personal care [18]. The Clinical Dementia Rating (CDR) has been standardized and implemented across various centers, including the Consortium to Establish a Registry for Alzheimer's Disease (CERAD) and the Alzheimer's Disease Cooperative Study, ensuring consistency in its application. Its reliability among different raters and validity in assessing dementia have been well-established. Additionally, the CDR has undergone neuropathological validation, particularly for determining the presence or absence of dementia. There are standardized training protocols available for its administration. While it may not be ideal for quick screening in population surveys due to the time required for interviews, the CDR is widely recognized in clinical settings as a dependable and valid global assessment tool for Alzheimer's disease.

The Clinical Dementia Rating Scale Sum of Boxes (CDR-SB) score is a tool used to assess the severity of dementia in clinical trials for Alzheimer's disease (Fig. 3). It

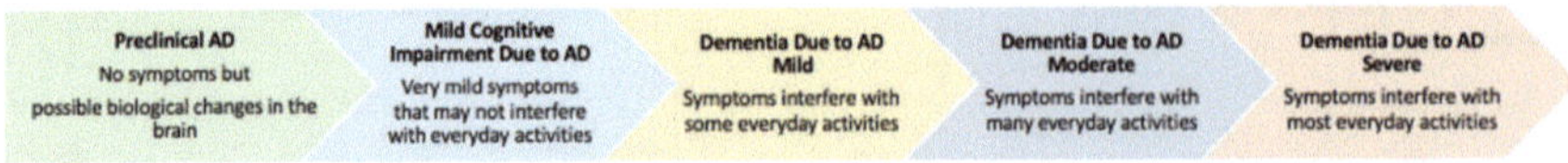

Fig. 3 Alzheimer's disease continuum [7]

Table 1 Clinical dementia rating [19]

Scale	Clinical dementia rating
0	Normal
0.5–4.0	Questionable cognitive impairment
0.5–2.5	Questionable impairment
3.0–4.0	Very mild dementia
4.5–9.0	Mild dementia
9.5–15.5	Moderate dementia
16.0–18.0	Severe dementia

is calculated by adding the ratings in each of the 6 categories of the scale. The score ranges from 0 to 18, with higher scores indicating greater impairment (Table 1).

4 Understanding Minimal Clinically Important Difference (MCID)

The minimal clinically important difference (MCID) is a term used to describe the smallest change in a treatment outcome that a patient would consider important. This change would be significant enough to warrant a change in the patient's management. The MCID score is a way to measure this change and is considered an attractive concept because it helps clinicians and researchers focus on patient-reported outcomes rather than just physical and radiological endpoints. It provides a threshold for determining whether an outcome is relevant to the patient, rather than just relying on statistical significance [20].

5 The Relation Between CDR and MCID

The Clinical Dementia Rating (CDR) Scale Sum of Boxes (SB) score is a valuable instrument employed in clinical trials to evaluate the level of dementia severity in individuals with Alzheimer's disease. Extensive research has been conducted to determine the minimal clinically important difference (MCID) for the CDR-SB score specifically in Alzheimer's patients. The findings indicated that a 1–2 point increase in the CDR-SB score corresponded to a significant decline in the patient's condition, representing a meaningful change. Moreover, the MCID values tended to escalate as the disease severity progressed [21].

6 Dementia in India

In India, there is a lack of effective social welfare programs that benefit people with dementia. The few programs that do exist are often plagued by corruption. While academic articles may discuss the issue, they provide little practical benefit to those affected by dementia, for lack of acceptance among other reasons.

Despite the diversity of cultures, religions, and socioeconomic statuses in India, there is a common trend of declining attention towards the elderly. Various studies have been conducted in India over years in this space. However, the studies have been restricted to regions and specific states, thus giving no clear estimate of this neurodegenerative disease. From various estimates, including sources such as Statista, we draw up a revised trend (Fig. 4), which issues an alarming increase in the prevalence and spread of dementia amongst the elderly. Emma Nichols et al. estimate the figure eleven million plus dementia patients in India (Table 2). However, we need to take into consideration that majority of the cases related to dementia go undetected in India. More so, we must also consider the priority treatment being given to other serious diseases including various types of Cancers, Diabetes, and Respiratory Diseases among others.

Increased lifespan adds to the dynamism even further with many associated diseases hitting the elderly population, leading to dementia at that age. One of the challenges faced in a country such as India is the issue of underdiagnosis of illness [22, 23]. We may also note that the cardiovascular diseases take the top spot amongst the leading contributors towards death or disability in India, and it is predicted that this would only increase in the coming decades [24]. According to an estimate, Alzheimer's and other types of dementias claimed 129,000 lives in India in 2019 [25]. The deaths due to Dementia and related diseases increased five time between 1990 and 2019.

Studies from countries across the globe suggest that early interventions such as changes in the diet, increased physical activity, and engaging the brain in writing and reading can reduce the risks of dementia. However, for these interventions to work in India, they must be tailored to the country's unique sociocultural environment [26], even though the essence of the activities would generally remain the same.

With no real figures of dementia available for Indian subcontinent, it becomes a real challenge for the researchers to work on prevention and cure of these neurogenerative disorders. A case in point is the estimates from two different sources and respective projections, as mentioned above. The difference between the projections works out to over 400%, which researchers may find difficult to contemplate. This creates a dissonance in the minds of the researchers and practitioners alike. Coupled with no clear cure for the disease, the patients are left to themselves, which forces them to consider alternate medicines such as Ayurveda and homeopathy.

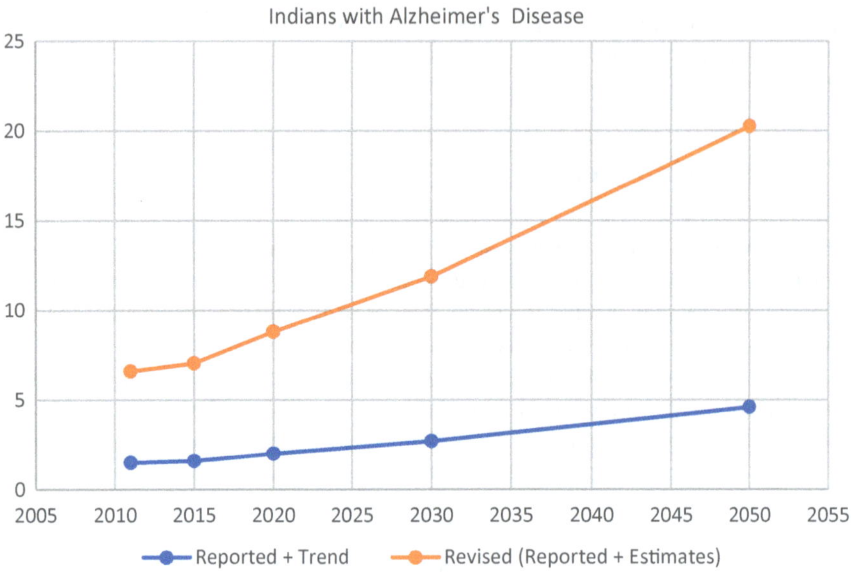

Fig. 4 Indians with Alzheimer's disease (Reported + Trend—[27]) and Revised Estimate (Author's own, based on various researches conducted in India; figures in millions

Table 2 An estimate by Nichols et al. [13]

India (Number of dementia cases in 2019 and 2050 and percentage change in counts and age-standardised rates)			
2019	2050	Counts	Age-standardised rates
38,43,118	11,422,692	197% (160 to 238)	6.4% (−3.6 to 20.4)

7 Developments in Treatment of Various Types of Dementia

With a wide range of challenges faced by the scientists, we have witnessed some position signs of finding a cure for Alzheimer's with potential use of insomnia drugs [28], which helps in blocking orexin with a dual orexin receptor antagonists (DORA) reduced levels of amyloid-β in the brain. These treatment is popularly known as anti-amyloid therapies [29]. Herbal medicine or Ayurveda, which originated in ancient cultures such as India, China and Egypt, uses specific medicinal plants to treat diseases and improve overall health. Many modern pharmaceuticals are based on synthesized versions of compounds found in plants. We have observed in recent times that there has been a renewed interest in ayurvedic/herbal medicines and its promise for treating diseases such as dementia, with minimal side effects. As one of the oldest forms of medicine, herbal remedies have been used by all cultures throughout history and their popularity continues to grow worldwide [30]. Probiotics have been reported for their efficacy to enhance memory [31]. Even as a single case does not get accepted for generalization of acceptance in the medical field, one of the cases that deserves a consideration is of a 70 plus year old female patient, who reported to a physiatrist with symptoms including insomnia, unconnected talking, irritation, weak memory & hygiene, and wandering away from home. She was diagnosed with dementia and given the homeopathic medicine Ignatia 200. Over a year, the patient's mini-mental state examination (MMSE[2]) score was revised from 10 (severe cognitive impairment) at baseline gradually improved to 24 (no cognitive impairment) [32]. Ignatia 200 is a homeopathic medicine used for depression and treating grief [33]. Another homeopathic medicine that has been strongly recommended for dementia patients is *Gingko* [34]. A simple search for the medicine on the internet states that this is a medicine for lowering of High Blood Pressure, lowering of burning sensation in chest and healing eruptions of cracks on the skin, thus creating a dissonance in the minds of the consumers. In short, there are homeopathic medicines only for prevention of the neurodegenerative diseases, and not a cure. We have a similar issue with herbal medicines. There's been research that concludes that music could be a powerful treatment strategy for dementia patients [35].

With the research in medicine science taking a new turn with an alternate use of drugs targeting the patients with attention-deficit hyperactivity disorder (ADHD), such as Adderall (amphetamine) and Ritalin (a stimulant for central nervous system) using the same for patients with various types of dementias could help.

In India, with a wider demographic profile, a divide between rural and urban regions, higher life expectancy and a relatively low literacy rate, alternative medicines have a better acceptance than the allopathic treatment in the rural areas. Add to this the cost factor and low levels of research (on a comparative state), and we have a dynamism that can, over time, create a state of an epidemic for the neurodegenerative disorder. The cost of such an epidemic will be huge for a developing economy such as India.

8 Treating Dementia in India

Since there are no major medical breakthroughs for treating dementia on the horizon, it's important to focus on preventing the disease. There are seven risk factors for Alzheimer's disease that can be modified: diabetes, midlife hypertension, midlife obesity, physical inactivity, depression, smoking, and low educational attainment. It is estimated that in India, 90% of people with dementia do not receive a diagnosis, treatment, or care for their condition [36]. This means that only 1 in 10 people

[2] The Mini-Mental State Examination (MMSE) is a short test that healthcare professionals use to measure cognitive impairment. It consists of a series of questions and tasks that assess various cognitive functions such as memory, language, and orientation. The test is scored out of 30 points, with a score of 25 or higher indicating normal cognitive function. The MMSE is a scientific tool used to measure cognitive impairment. It is widely used in both clinical and research settings and has been shown to be a valid and reliable way to diagnose and track the progression of Alzheimer's disease.

with dementia in India are receiving the help they need. Depressive symptoms were reported by 31% of older adults living in rural areas and 27% of those living in urban areas [37]. The mental health of older adults is affected by factors such as geriatric depression, insomnia and other sleep issues, and social isolation. These issues highlight the importance of paying attention to this demographic [10]. By reducing the prevalence of these risk factors by 10% per decade, it's estimated that the prevalence of Alzheimer's disease could be reduced by 8.3% worldwide by 2050 [38].

Improving access to education and targeting vascular risk factors and depression can also help reduce the incidence of Alzheimer's disease. In 2010 it was estimated that the total cost of dementia in India was US$ 3.415 billion (INR 147 billion), with 56% of that cost being for informal care and 29% for direct medical costs [39]. There has been no recent study in this area. The annual cost of caring for a person with dementia in India varies depending on the severity of the disease and whether the person lives in an urban or rural area. In urban areas, the cost ranges from INR 45,600 to INR 2,02,450 while in rural areas it ranges from INR 20,300 to INR 66,025 [39]. However, with an average inflation of 5% pa, we can only expect this cost to move upwards. Since there's no clear treatment available for dementia, the medicines available and prevalent in India are targeted for temporarily improvement of the symptoms but not as a cure. On an average, the cost is about Rs. 8,000 per month for allopathic treatment and around Rs. 10,000 for ayurvedic medicines. As we can observe, the care cost is higher when compared to the medicines.

9 Conclusion

As family sizes decrease, single children and grandchildren may find it difficult to care for their elderly relatives. Dementia care has already impacted general health-care. Prior to the pandemic, up to a quarter of beds in hospitals were occupied by dementia patients [40]. It is imperative for governments to take immediate action to mitigate the social and economic consequences of the rising prevalence of dementia. To begin, it is crucial to acknowledge the sense of urgency that was expressed by many just a few years ago. We may note that the funding for dementia research has significantly lagged behind that of cancer or coronary heart disease [40]. The governments must consider the provision of long-term care for individuals with dementia, especially when we have observed a drop in the family size across developing and developed countries, which directly impact the caring of the elderly. The most important concern of financing such care of dementia patients. While Japan's compulsory long-term care insurance scheme, which mandates individuals aged 40–65 to pay a premium, appears appealing as it avoids penalizing younger generations, it may not be financially self-sustaining. As the burden continues to increase, it is imperative that the responsibility of funding will ultimately fall upon individuals and taxpayers. And a question even more fundamental than who will finance the care is: who will provide it? Providing care for individuals with dementia, with compassion and dignity, requires a significant amount of labour. While technology can assist in alleviating some of the burden by enabling remote monitoring and potentially utilizing robots for basic tasks in the future, the core of dementia care revolves around human interaction. Unfortunately, this occupation is often classified as low-skilled and receives inadequate compensation. In reality, it demands immense reserves of patience, empathy, and kindness. It should be recognized as a more valuable profession and rewarded accordingly, despite the potential increase in costs. Countries such as Japan and Britain, facing severe shortages of care workers, may need to ease immigration policies to attract individuals who are willing and capable of fulfilling these roles. Furthermore, evidence suggests that up to 40% of dementia cases can be delayed or prevented by adopting healthy behaviours earlier in life. However, public health campaigns in this regard have had mixed results, and they do not address dementia's most stubborn pre-existing condition—old age [40]. Without a cure, insufficient funding, and the complexities of conveying a public health message, it may seem tempting to feel despair and give up. Nevertheless, these challenges only emphasize that the solutions for dementia, much like the disease itself, will require decades to unfold. This realization serves as another compelling reason to commence working on these solutions immediately.

References

1. Oh, E. S., & Rabins, P. V. (2019). Dementia. *Annals of Internal Medicine, 171*, ITC33–ITC48. https://doi.org/10.7326/AITC201909030
2. Srivastava, S., Ahmad, R., & Khare, S. K. (2021). Alzheimer's disease and its treatment by different approaches: A review. *European Journal of Medicinal Chemistry, 216*, 113320. https://doi.org/10.1016/j.ejmech.2021.113320
3. Lyketsos, C. G., Carrillo, M. C., Ryan, J. M., Khachaturian, A. S., Trzepacz, P., Amatniek, J., et al. (2011). Neuropsychiatric symptoms in Alzheimer's disease. *Alzheimer's Dementia, 7*, 532–539. https://doi.org/10.1016/j.jalz.2011.05.2410
4. Gao, Y., & Liu, X. (2021). Secular trends in the incidence of and mortality due to Alzheimer's disease and other forms of dementia in China From 1990 to 2019: An age-period-cohort study and joinpoint analysis. *Frontiers in Aging Neuroscience, 13*, 709156. https://doi.org/10.3389/fnagi.2021.709156
5. Lee, J., Meijer, E., Langa, K. M., et al. (2023). Prevalence of dementia in India: National and state estimates from a nationwide study. *Alzheimer's Dementia*, 1–15. https://doi.org/10.1002/alz.12928
6. WHO, World Health Organization. (2023). https://www.who.int/news-room/fact-sheets/detail/dementia#:~:text=Key%20facts,nearly%2010%20million%20new%20cases.
7. ADI, Alzheimer's Disease International. (2023). https://www.alzint.org/about/dementia-facts-figures/dementia-statistics/
8. Hou, Y., Dan, X., Babbar, M. et al. (2019). Ageing as a risk factor for neurodegenerative disease. *Nature Reviews Neurology, 15*, 565–581. https://doi.org/10.1038/s41582-019-0244-7
9. Wyss-Coray, T. (2016). Ageing, neurodegeneration and brain rejuvenation. *Nature, 539*, 180–186.
10. Arora, A. (2023). The Mint, We need to talk about the mental health of seniors. https://epaper.livemint.com/Home/ArticleView?utm_source=LM_Desk_Header&utm_medium=LM_desk_top_nav&utm_campaign=Ref

11. Li, X., Feng, X., Sun, X., Hou, N., Han, F., & Liu, Y. (2022). Global, regional, and national burden of Alzheimer's disease and other dementias, 1990–2019. *Frontiers in Aging Neuroscience, 14*, 937486. https://doi.org/10.3389/fnagi.2022.937486
12. Mouches, P., Langner, S., Domin, M., Hill, M. D., & Forkert, N. D. (2021). Influence of cardiovascular risk-factors on morphological changes of cerebral arteries in healthy adults across the life span. *Scientific Reports, 11*, 12236.
13. Nichols, E., Steinmetz, J. D., Vollset, S. E., Fukutaki, K., Chalek, J., Abd-Allah, F., Abdoli, A., Abualhasan, A., Abu-Gharbieh, E., Tayyaba Akram, T., Al Hamad, H., Alahdab, F., Alanezi, F. M., Alipour, V., Almustanyir, S., Amu, H., Ansari, I., Arabloo, J., Ashraf, T., & Astell-Burt, T. et al. (2022). Estimation of the global prevalence of dementia in 2019 and forecasted prevalence in 2050: an analysis for the Global Burden of Disease Study 2019. *The Lancet Public Health, 7*(2), e105–e125. ISSN 2468–2667. https://doi.org/10.1016/S2468-2667(21)00249-8
14. Mantri, S., Fullard, M., Gray, S. L., Weintraub, D., Hubbard, R. A., Hennessy, S., & Willis, A. W. (2019). Patterns of dementia treatment and frank prescribing errors in older adults with Parkinson disease. *JAMA neurology, 76*(1), 41–49. https://doi.org/10.1001/jamaneurol.2018.2820
15. Bhattacharyya, K. K. (2021). Aging and dementia. In *Rethinking the aging transition*. Springer. https://doi.org/10.1007/978-3-030-88870-1_7
16. Lustig, C., & Lin, Z. (2016). Memory: Behavior and neural basis. In K. W. Schaie & S. L. Willis (Eds.), *Handbook of the psychology of aging* (8th edn, pp. 147–163). Academic Press.
17. Knopman, D. S., & Petersen, R. C. (2014). Mild cognitive impairment and mild dementia: A clinical perspective. *Mayo Clinic Proceedings, 89*(10), 1452–1459. https://doi.org/10.1016/j.mayocp.2014.06.019
18. Morris, J. (1997). Clinical dementia rating: A reliable and valid diagnostic and staging measure for dementia of the Alzheimer type. *International Psychogeriatrics, 9*(S1), 173–176. https://doi.org/10.1017/S1041610297004870
19. Caselli, R. J., & Boeve, B. F. (2007). Chapter 33—the degenerative dementias. In Goetz, C. G. (Eds.), *Textbook of clinical neurology* (3rd edn, pp. 699–733). W.B. Saunders. ISBN 9781416036180. https://doi.org/10.1016/B978-141603618-0.10033-5.
20. Wright, A., Hannon, J., Hegedus, E. J., & Kavchak, A. E. (2012). Clinimetrics corner: A closer look at the minimal clinically important difference (MCID). *The Journal of Manual & Manipulative Therapy, 20*(3), 160–166. https://doi.org/10.1179/2042618612Y.0000000001.PMID:23904756;PMCID:PMC3419574
21. Andrews, J. S., Desai, U., Kirson, N. Y., Zichlin, M. L., Ball, D. E., & Matthews, B. R. (2019). Disease severity and minimal clinically important differences in clinical outcome assessments for Alzheimer's disease clinical trials. *Alzheimer's & Dementia: Translational Research & Clinical Interventions, 5*, 354–363. ISSN 2352-8737. https://doi.org/10.1016/j.trci.2019.06.005
22. Claypool, K. T., Chung, M. K., Deonarine, A., Gregg, E. W., & Patel, C. J. (2020). Characteristics of undiagnosed diabetes in men and women under the age of 50 years in the Indian subcontinent: The National Family Health Survey (NFHS-4)/demographic health survey 2015–2016. *BMJ Open Diabetes Research and Care*, 8, e000965.
23. Prenissl, J., et al. (2019). Hypertension screening, awareness, treatment, and control in India: A nationally representative cross-sectional study among individuals aged 15 to 49 years. *PLoS Medicine, 16*, e1002801.
24. Patel, V., et al. (2011). Chronic diseases and injuries in India. *Lancet, 377*, 413–428.
25. Samreen, V. (2022). *Alzheimer's-related deaths in India increased 5 times in 30 years*. Business Standard. https://www.business-standard.com/article/current-affairs/alzheimer-s-related-deaths-in-india-increased-5-times-in-30-years-122100300571_1.html
26. Ravindranath, V., & Sundarakumar, J. S. (2021). Changing demography and the challenge of dementia in India. *Nature Reviews Neurology, 17*, 747–758. https://doi.org/10.1038/s41582-021-00565-x
27. Statista. (2020). APA, Chicago, Harvard, MLA & Bluebook. https://www.statista.com/statistics/944170/india-number-of-cases-of-alzheimer-s-disease-in-senior-citizens/

28. NIA, National Institute of Ageing. (2023). https://www.nia.nih.gov/news/insomnia-drug-may-lower-levels-alzheimers-proteins
29. Wired. (2023). https://www.wired.com/story/alzheimers-drugs-benefits-risks-lecanemab-donanemab/
30. Akram, M., & Nawaz, A. (2017). Effects of medicinal plants on Alzheimer's disease and memory deficits. *Neural Regeneration Research, 12*(4), 660–670. https://doi.org/10.4103/1673-5374.205108.PMID:28553349;PMCID:PMC5436367
31. Lyte, M. (2011). Probiotics function mechanistically as delivery vehicles for neuroactive compounds: Microbial endocrinology in the design and use of probiotics. *BioEssays, 33*, 74–81.
32. Gilla, D., Devasia, M. N., L AA. (2022), Dementia treated with individualized homoeopathy: A case report. *Indian Journal of Research in Homoeopathy*, *16*(2), 10. Available from: https://ijrh.researchcommons.org/journal/vol16/iss2/10
33. Healthline. (2016). https://www.healthline.com/health/can-ignatia-help-anxiety
34. Homeopathy360. https://www.homeopathy360.com/2020/06/26/alzheimers-disease-and-homoeopathy-2/
35. Moreno-Morales, C., Calero, R., Moreno-Morales, P., Pintado, C. (2020). Music therapy in the treatment of dementia: A systematic review and meta-analysis. *Frontiers in Medicine.* https://doi.org/10.3389/fmed.2020.00160
36. Nulkar, A., Paralikar, V., & Juvekar, S. (2019). Dementia in India—a call for action. *Journal of Global Health Reports., 3*, e2019078. https://doi.org/10.29392/joghr.3.e2019078
37. Hossain, B., Nagargoje, V. P., Sk, M. I. K. et al. (2022). Social exclusion and mental health among older adults: cross-sectional evidence from a population-based survey in India. *BMC Psychiatry*, *22*, 409. https://doi.org/10.1186/s12888-022-04064-1
38. Kumar, C. T., George, S., & Kallivayalil, R. A. (2019). Towards a dementia-friendly India. *Indian Journal of Psychological Medicine, 41*, 476–481.
39. Rao, G. N., & Bharath, S. (2013). Cost of dementia care in India: Delusion or reality? *Indian Journal of Public Health, 57*, 71–77.
40. The Economist. (2020). https://www.economist.com/leaders/2020/08/27/the-rising-prevalence-of-dementia-is-a-global-emergency

Exploring AI's Role in Managing Neurodegenerative Disorders: Possibilities and Hurdles

Sudheer Mangalampalli, Ganesh Reddy Karri, and Aditi Shaw

Abstract Neurodegenerative diseases are an ever-growing type of a disease which is very common in elderly people. With the increase in the population of older people (aged 65 and above), these diseases have increased in number by a considerable rate. Currently there is no cure for neurodegenerative diseases. A patient who has developed one of these diseases is diagnosed and given certain medications which can help them to slow down the symptoms, but the diseases are incurable. The diseases include Alzheimer's disease, Parkinson's disease, Lewy body dementia, frontotemporal disease, multiple sclerosis, amyotrophic lateral sclerosis, Huntington's disease, Chromatic Traumatic Encephalopathy, progressive supranuclear palsy and others. These diseases include various symptoms like depression, anxiety, losing control over muscle movement, degradation in performance, eventually depending on others for daily tasks, difficulty in remembering things and several other symptoms. Diagnosing these diseases is a long and tedious method and it requires a lot of money. Identification of these type of diseases is itself a big task and different expensive tests like CT scan and MRI scan are prescribed to the patients to find out the type of biomarker present in their brain. After analysis the type of biomarker and why the nerve cells in the brain and the spinal cord are degrading, doctors conclude about the type of disease a patient might be suffering from. Several drugs are prescribed to the patients based on their condition. One type of a drug may not suit two patients suffering from the same type of disease. Hence, finding out the type of disease a patient is going through along with the type of medicine that might suit them is not an easy task. Hence, with the help of AI, researchers are trying to find ways to diagnose and prescribe the patients in an easy, cost-effective manner with less invasiveness. Machine Learning model like Random Forest comes handy when trying to identify the type of marker present in the brain cells of the patients. With the help of the already existing datasets along with the diagnosis data of the patient, the model can easily predict about the type of biomarker present thereby giving an easy and mostly accurate result about the type of biomarker present. Random forest algorithm, along with deep learning modules is helping to predict and give faster and accurate

S. Mangalampalli (✉) · G. R. Karri · A. Shaw
School of Computer Science and Engineering, VIT-AP University, Amaravati, Andhra Pradesh, India
e-mail: sudheerkietmtech@gmail.com

© The Author(s), under exclusive license to Springer Nature Switzerland AG 2024

L. Gaur et al. (eds.), *AI and Neuro-Degenerative Diseases*, Studies in Computational Intelligence 1131, https://doi.org/10.1007/978-3-031-53148-4_7

results on the type of diseases. These models are rigorously being trained with every time new datasets being added, which gives us more accurate results. With the help of AI, automated drug prediction for patients, early diagnosis, biomarker prediction, course and progression of a disease can be predicted easily and with the advancement in research, AI is proving to be promising enough so become more and more efficient and reliable. Using AI in the field of neurodegenerative diseases has made it a lot easier to monitor the diseases and help deal with them in a better manner. Using Ensemble based models and ADNI databases which offers multi-modal data, makes it easier for AI to predict neurodegenerative diseases at an early stage, find the diseases' course and progression, and also prescribe the patients with the type of drugs that will suit their body. However, as there as many opportunities to use AI in the field of neurodegenerative diseases, it also has its own challenges.

1 Introduction

1.1 What Are Neurodegenerative Diseases?

Neurodegenerative diseases, also known as degenerative nerve diseases, are symptoms that affect how the entire human body works [1]. These diseases gradually damage the parts of our nervous system, especially our brain [2]. It involves the death of nerve cells in brain or peripheral nervous system because of the nerve cells losing its functionalities. These diseases are said to more likely develop in elderly population. Recent researches have shown that there is an increase in the number of neurodegenerative diseases with the increase in the population of elderly people (aged 65 and older). These diseases develop slowly and start showing symptoms gradually over time. It is said that once a person develops a neurodegenerative disease, it just grows and the rate of growth can be slowed down but not stopped. These diseases are considered as incurable (Fig. 1).

1.2 Types of Neurodegenerative Diseases

The term "neurodegenerative diseases" does not specify only one type of a disease, but it defines a vast set of diseases that fall under this term [2, 3]. Types of neurodegenerative diseases include: Alzheimer's disease, Parkinson's disease, Huntington's disease, Multiple sclerosis, Amyotrophic lateral sclerosis, progressive supranuclear palsy (PSP), Creutzfeldt-Jakob disease, frontotemporal dementia, chronic traumatic encephalopathy (CTE), Huntington's disease, Lewy body dementia and several others.

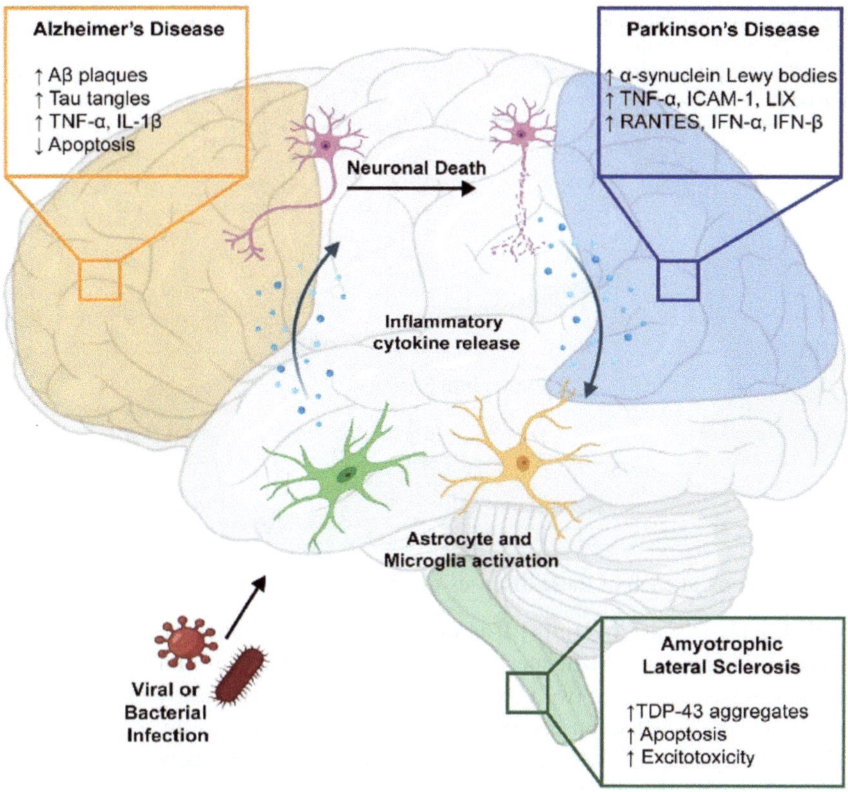

Fig. 1 Different parts of the brain that are affected by different types of neurodegenerative diseases [2]

The above listed diseases are sub-grouped into different types of diseases as:

- **Dementia type diseases**: These include Alzheimer's disease, frontotemporal disease, chronic traumatic encephalopathy (CTE) and Lewy body dementia. These diseases affect certain brain areas and includes death of neurons.
- **Parkinsonism type diseases**: This includes Parkinson's disease and other forms of Parkinsonism. These diseases affect neurons that helps with body coordination and precise control or muscle movements.
- **Demyelinating diseases**: Includes multiple sclerosis, and others. These diseases tend to damage myelin which affects the sending and relaying of nerve signals.
- **Motor Neuron diseases**: Includes Amyotrophic lateral sclerosis, also called as "Lou Gehrig's disease" and progressive supranuclear palsy (PSP). These diseases are caused when the neurons that control movement dies.
- **Prion diseases**: A type of protein misfolding disease, causing severe damage in a short period of time, commonly including Creutzfeldt-Jakob disease, which happens for unknown reasons.

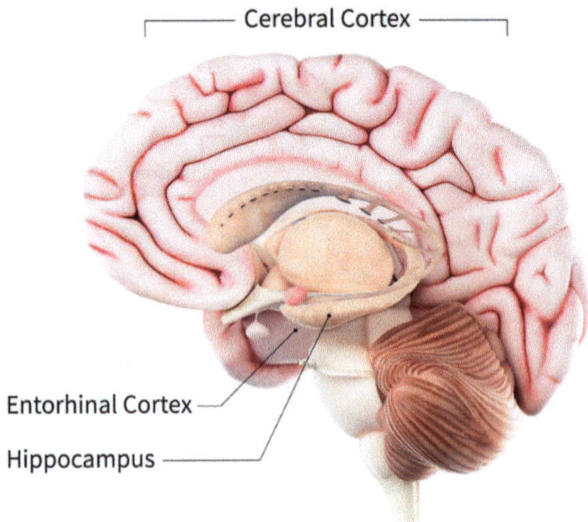

Fig. 2 Entorhinal cortex and hippocampus of the brain gets affected by Alzheimer's disease [5]

Let us look at each of these diseases in details:

Alzheimer's Disease (AD): [4] It is one of the most common neurodegenerative diseases. People with Alzheimer's disease lose the ability to think and carry out simplest tasks. There are two types of Alzheimer's disease—early-onset type and late-onset type. The late-onset type AD is more common and it affects people above 65 years of age. Early-onset type AD is more common in people between ages 30 and 65. It affects the neurons in several parts of the brain. There is no effective treatment for Alzheimer's disease yet (Fig. 2).

Common symptoms include:

- personality loss
- getting lost
- Change in personality
- Language problems

Frontotemporal Disease: [6] This disease is associated with affecting parts of the frontal lobe of the brain. Personality, behavior, and language changes are the problems faced by patients diagnosed with frontotemporal disease [7]. Frontotemporal dementia occurs usually from age between 40 and 65 and constitute nearly 10%–20% of the total dementia cases (Fig. 3).

Common symptoms include:

- Loss of empathy
- Lack of judgement
- Lack of interest
- Muscle problems
- Falls or walking problems
- Forgetting meaning of words etc.

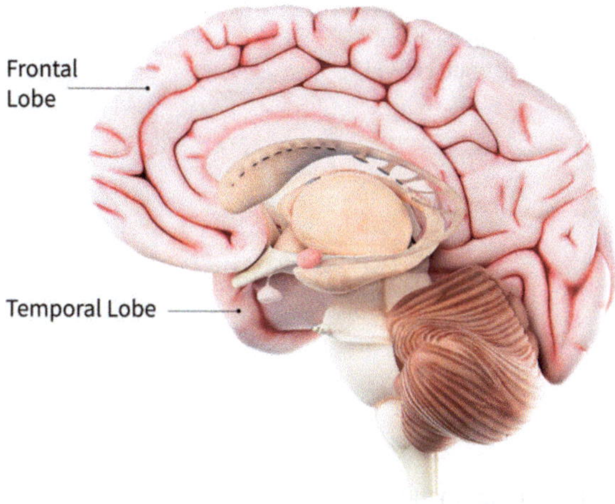

Fig. 3 Frontal lobe of the brain gets affected due to degeneration of nerve cells [8]

Chronic Traumatic Encephalopathy (CTE):

[9] Occurs in people who get repeatedly injured in their head. There is no prominent explanation about this disease and it is rare in the case of degenerative diseases [10]. This mostly occurs when the head gets injured before it recovers from the previously head injury, also known as second impact syndrome (Fig. 4).

Common symptoms include:

- Impulsive behavior
- Aggression

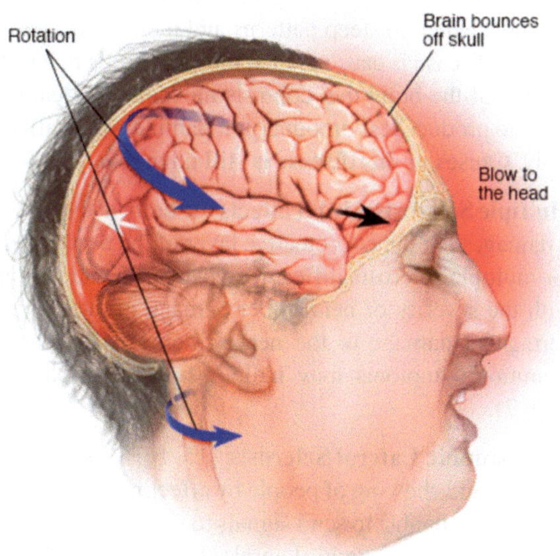

Fig. 4 Brain getting affected by chronic traumatic encephalopathy because of frequent head injuries [11]

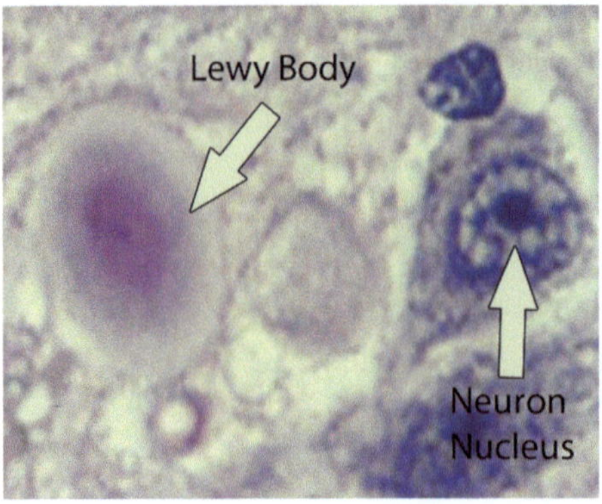

Fig. 5 Lewy body accumulating in the brain and affecting brain cells [13]

- Emotional instability etc.

Lewy Body Dementia: This is the second most common neurodegenerative disease after Alzheimer's disease [12]. In this disease, a type of protein deposit called Lewy body is built up on the nerve cells, which impacts several actions of the body. It can cause Parkinson's disease symptoms in people (Fig. 5).

Parkinson's Disease: It is a brain disorder that causes the body to act in an uncontrollable way. Such as shaking of body, lack in body balance and coordination, body stiffness etc. It occurs in people above 60 years of age. However, 5%–10% of the people suffering from Parkinson's disease experience the onset before the age of 50. Studies show that this disease affect more men than women. The affects of Parkinson's disease worsen over time and gradually, patients diagnosed with Parkinson's disease develop difficulty in walking and talking. Over time, patients suffer with depression, fatigue, change in sleep patterns and memory difficulties.

This disease is caused when the nerve cells in basal ganglia dies. Basal ganglia is an area of the brain that controls movements. Death of these nerve cells causes the brain to produce less amount of dopamine which affects the overall movement of the body. Causes of this disease is still unknown (Fig. 6).

Multiple Sclerosis: [14] It affects the brain and spinal cord (central nervous system). It damages the upper protective layer of the nerve fibers called as myelin. Symptoms for multiple sclerosis differ from patient to patient depending on the location along with the severity of nerve fiber damage in the spinal cord. This disease can cause permanent damage to the nerve fiber, i.e., the damage process is not reversible. Common symptoms may include numbness, pain and tickling in parts of body (Fig. 7).

Amyotrophic Lateral Sclerosis: [15, 16] This neurodegenerative disease affects the walking and chewing of people by affecting the motor neurons. As a result, the motor neurons are unable to send signals to the muscles to help them function a certain way. The cause of amyotrophic lateral sclerosis may include smoking, environmental toxin exposure and military service. The chances of having diagnosed with ALS is higher

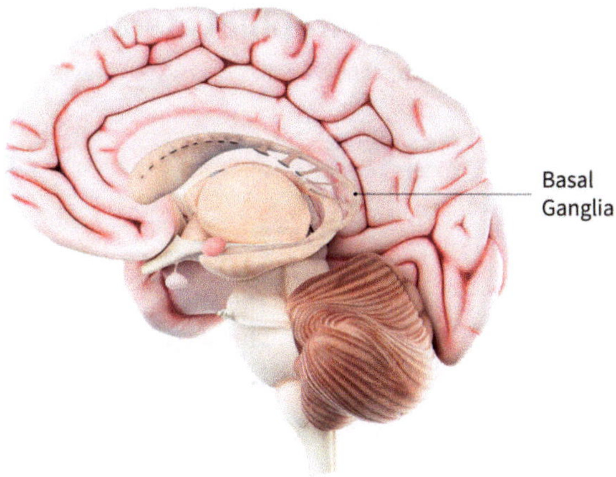

Fig. 6 Nerve cells in basal ganglia dies leading to Parkinson's disease [11]

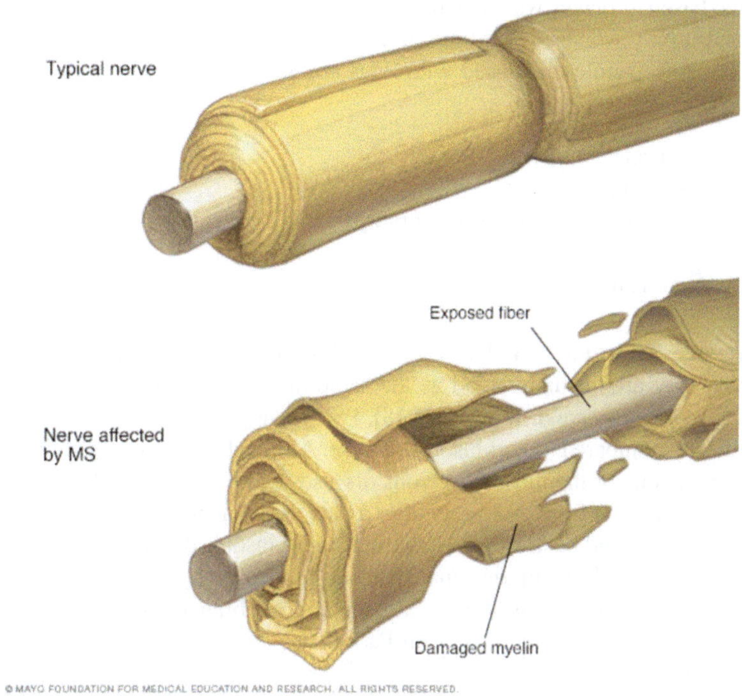

Fig. 7 Myelin getting damaged by multiple sclerosis [9]

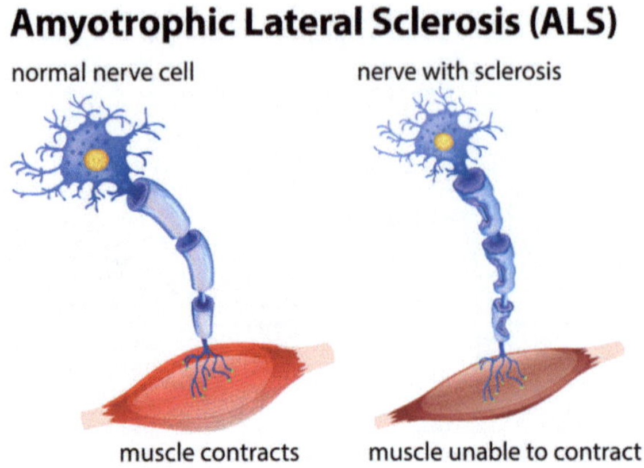

Fig. 8 Nerve cell losing its ability to control muscle movement because of damage [12]

in women compared to that in men. This disease is also called as Lou Gehrig's disease after the baseball player who was diagnosed with this disease. There is no cure for ALS and it only worsens over time. It can also be considered as a genetic disease as nearly 10% people diagnosed with ALS are genetic cases. Common symptoms include (Fig. 8):

- Loss of muscle control
- Slurred speeches
- Weakness in muscles and muscle cramps
- Tripping and falling
- Emotional disbalance etc.

Progressive Supranuclear Palsy (PSP): PSP is like Parkinson's disease, but however, they are misunderstood as the same disease. Although both are similar, but the two diseases are different [17, 18]. PSP occurs in the mid to late 60's, which is much later compared to Parkinson's disease. Although the two have similar symptoms, PSP is one of the most dangerous diseases and it can cause almost complete inability in a person from 3–5 years after a person is diagnosed with it [18]. In PSP, patients tend to bend backwards. However, in Parkinson's disease, the patients tend to bend forwards. The symptoms in PSP are also much stronger and identified earlier compared to Parkinson's disease. In PSP, the affected brain cells are accumulated in the form of a protein called as tau. In Parkinson's disease, the protein is called as alpha-synuclein (Fig. 9).

Creutzfeldt-Jakob Disease: [19] This is one the most dangerous type of neurodegenerative disease and patients diagnosed with this are most likely to die within one year after the onset of the disease. This disease does not have a cure and it spreads very rapidly. This disease is believed to happen by prion protein, which is an abnormal isoform of a cellular glycoprotein. As this is also a neurodegenerative disease, the symptoms are almost similar to those of the other mentioned diseases. But, CJD has two main symptoms and these include:

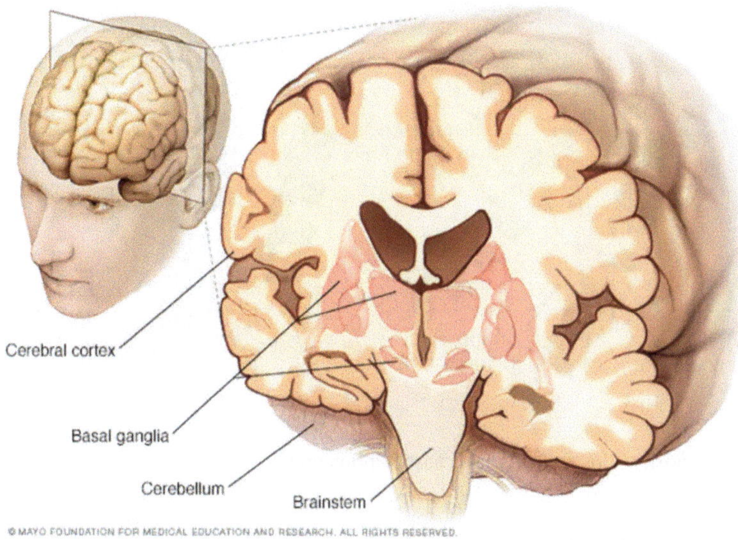

Fig. 9 Deterioration of nerve cells in the brainstem, cerebral cortex, cerebellum and basal ganglia [13]

1. Unwanted muscle movement
2. Extreme mental collapsing and dementia

Early symptoms of CJD includes behavioral changes, depression and anxiety, vision changes, lack of balance and coordination and Insomnia. As the disease progresses, we can see symptoms like blindness, coma, arms and legs becoming weak and losing the ability to speak.

There are several ways to diagnose CJD but as of now, there is no cure for the disease. This disease is similar to Alzheimer's and Huntington's disease which also worsen over time and have no cure (Fig. 10).

Huntington's Disease: It is one of the rare neurodegenerative diseases and is genetic. Symptoms develop in a person's 30's or 40's. However, in rare cases, the symptoms may also arise in early 20's and is called as juvenile Huntington's Disease. It has a great impact on muscle movement, thinking and mental disorders. The disease develops faster in patients who are diagnosed with it at a younger age. The symptoms of Huntington's disease differ from that of juvenile Huntington's Disease.

Common symptoms of Huntington's disease include:

- Muscle problems
- Unwanted movement of muscles
- Unusual eye movement
- Problems with speech
- Lack of impulse control
- Lack of organization

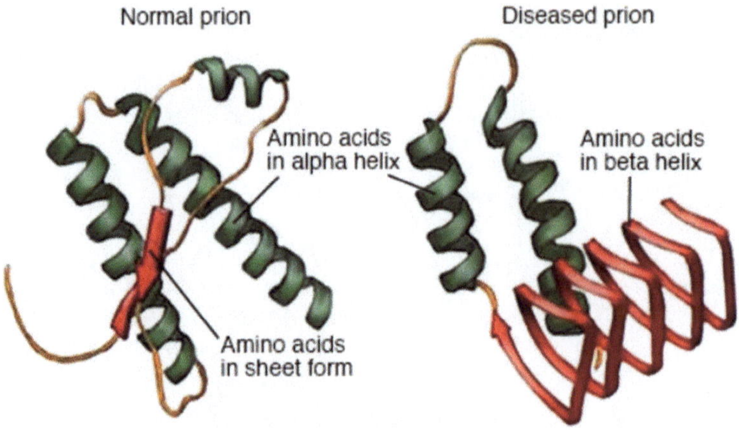

Fig. 10 Amino acids losing its form because of prion protein [9]

- Difficulty in learning something new
- Fatigue
- Insomnia
- Social isolation

Common symptoms of juvenile Huntington's disease include (Fig. 11):

- Difficulty in paying attention
- Behavioral changes
- Significant drop in performance related to school or work
- Slight unwanted muscular movement
- Seizures.

1.3 Symptoms of Neurodegenerative Diseases

[20] So, to summarize some of the most important neurodegenerative diseases discussed above, we can list the symptoms of these diseases as the following:

- Change in thinking patterns
- Losing balance and control
- Weakening eyesight
- Emotional instability
- Loss of muscle control
- Memory loss
- Depression and anxiety
- Unwanted thoughts
- Longer amount of time required to learn new skills

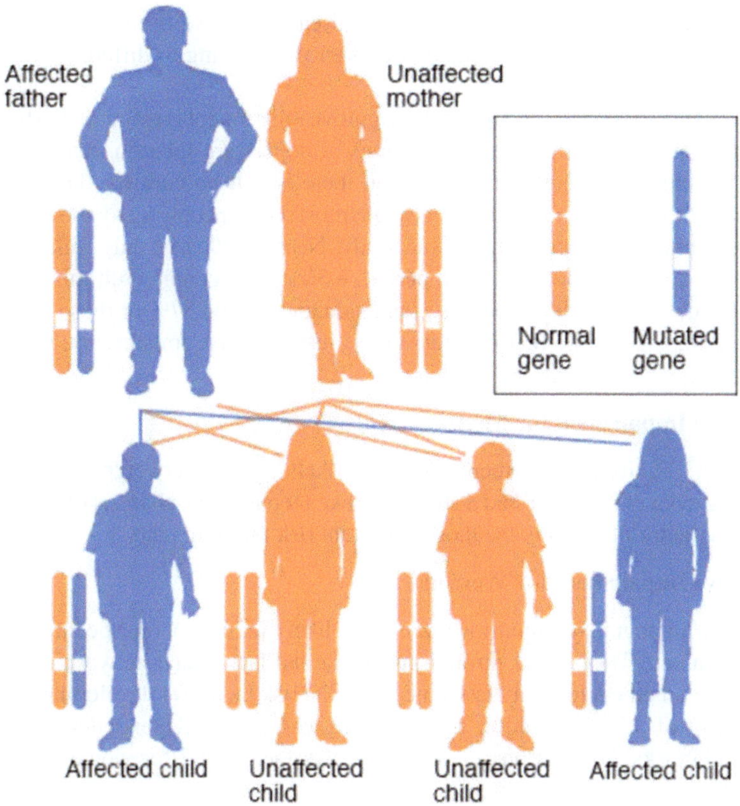

Fig. 11 Showing the genetic mutation of Huntington's disease [14]

People who feel the symptoms mentioned above should immediately consult a doctor to recognize the diseases at the early stage. To find if a person is suffering from a neurodegenerative disease, the doctor first checks the patient's cognitive function.

[11, 21] Cognitive functions are mental abilities such as learning, thinking, problem solving, remembering things, decision making and attention. If a person lacks these abilities, then the doctor might recommend an MRI scan to confirm the diagnosis. To find the presence of microRNAs, a test is recommended, since microRNAs contain potential biomarkers to identify if the patient is suffering from neurodegenerative disease.

1.4 Gender Matters for Cognitive Impairment Risk

It is interesting to note that these diseases affect men and women differently. Cognitive impairment is basically the loss of brain functionalities. Gender makes a huge difference in diagnosing neurodegenerative diseases as these diseases affect men and women differently. These risk factors are varied according to different age groups for men and women.

According to statistics, people with cognitive impairment is estimated to be nearly 13.2 million by 2050 in US alone. Billions of dollars are spent in treating patients with Alzheimer's and other dementia but there is still no cure for these diseases. According to a study in France including almost 7,000 people aged above 65; none had dementia at the beginning of the study. Nearly 42% had only mild cognitive impairment. Over a four-year time period, 6.5% of the people with mild cognitive impairment saw that they developed dementia and around 37% of those returned to normal. So, we can see that if a person has just cognitive impairment, that can be revered.

Cognitive Impairment for Men

Men with cognitive impairment are more likely to be overweight and might be suffering from diabetes, or had a stroke. Stroke increases the chances of dementia in men by a factor of 3 and is the most important risk factor in men.

Cognitive Impairment for Women

Women with cognitive impairment are more likely to have poorer health and physically disabled. They suffer through insomnia and lack social network. A woman, dependent on others for daily tasks increases the risk factor for developing dementia by a factor of 3.5 compared to those women who are not dependent on others for their daily tasks. Depressions increases the risk factor by 2 for women to develop dementia.

Why is Cognitive Impairment Different for Men and Women?

There is no particular or correct answer as to why the cognitive impairment differs in men and women. What has been found from the studies is that, men are affected by physical health and women are more related to relationship-based criteria for developing dementia.

Can Cognitive Impairment Be Avoided or Reduced?

There is no evidence to prove that cognitive impairment can be avoided or reduced, but one can follow some of the mentioned practices to sustain as healthy life:

- Preventing smoking
- Managing diabetes
- Maintaining a healthy weight
- Maintaining good relationships
- Preventing and treating depression.

1.5 Causes of Neurodegenerative Diseases

As we have discussed, age is the most important risk factor in neurodegenerative disease and it is always associated with some risk factors. Aging causes the nerve cells of the brain and the central nervous system to slow down and eventually die. Pathogenic proteins are accumulated which causes different types of neurodegenerative diseases. These diseases can also be genetic and affect men and women differently.

The following can be some of the causes of neurodegenerative diseases:

Neuronal Damage

Neurodegenerative diseases are caused when the nerve cells in the brain and spinal cord are damaged. As the age of a man progresses, these diseases cause more and more nerve cells to die leading to inability to move, speak, think etc. As the age gets older, the brain shrinks, and the dead nerve cells cannot replace itself with newer nerve cells.

Environmental Factors

Environment and surroundings can also have a great impact on the onset of the diseases. Exposure to certain toxins in the environment, or dealing with certain chemicals can cause certain pathogenic growth in the central nervous system, which can lead the brain cells to get affected and eventually die.

Genetic Factors

The neurogenerative diseases can be genetic too. Passing down of mutated genes can cause certain neurodegenerative diseases to develop inside the body. Environmental and genetic factors combined causes several neurodegenerative conditions.

Abnormal Proteins

Presence of abnormal proteins in the brain like Lewy bodies, prion protein, tau, synuclein, beta-amyloid etc., causes the nerve cells in the brain to die, thereby leading to several diseases.

Other than the above-mentioned causes, these diseases can also be caused by other factors like:

- Smoking
- Poor diet
- Obesity
- Stroke
- Depression
- Alcoholism
- Tumor.

1.6 Treatments for Neurodegenerative Diseases

Till date, there is no cure for degenerative diseases. These diseases, after their onset, can only grow. However, with time, science and its advancement in technology has led us to find several solutions to better understand the diseases [22]. Development and testing of new treatments are still an ongoing process and currently there are no known cures for neurodegenerative disease.

Alzheimer's Disease: In the recent years, with the enhancement in studies for Alzheimer's disease, we have got to know that administration (FDA) approved drugs [23] are best suited for people diagnosed with early stages of Alzheimer's. However, any one drug, as mentioned earlier is not suitable for all the patients who are suffering through Alzheimer's [24]. For mild to moderate Alzheimer's, drugs like rivastigmine, galantamine and donepezil are prescribed. All of these drugs are cholinesterase inhibitors which will help to reduce or control cognitive symptoms. These inhibitors prevent acetylcholine from breaking down, which is considered as an important chemical for memory. However, these inhibitors can just inhibit the growth of the disease and cannot completely stop it. FDA approved immunotherapies, lecanemab and aducanumab have been effective in reducing amyloid plaques, but they still can't prove to reduce cognitive decline rate. For moderate to severe Alzheimer's, memantine is used to decrease the symptoms. These drugs can only reduce the effects of Alzheimer's and help patients to work independently for maybe a few more months. There is no proper cure for Alzheimer's.

Frontotemporal Disease: Identifying frontotemporal disease might be a little bit problematic as its conditions can overlap with those of liver or kidney disease. So, a blood test is recommended to know the situation of liver and kidney. Sleeping patterns are tested and studies along with memory-based tests. MRI scans and FDG-PET scans are also done to check the metabolism of nutrient content in parts of brain. As mentioned earlier, there is no cure for these diseases and the drugs used in Alzheimer's are not used for frontotemporal disease. Antidepressants and antipsychotics like citalopram, paroxetine or sertraline, and olanzapine or quetiapine are found effective in this type of disease.

Chronic Traumatic Encephalopathy (CTE): There are no known drugs that can help a patient suffering from chronic traumatic encephalopathy, and the conditions just keep on worsening over time. However, a clinical criterion has been developed for traumatic encephalopathy syndrome (TES), which is associated with CTE. Evidence for deposits of tau and other proteins in the brain, along with the degradation of nerve cells are required to diagnose the patient which can only be done during an autopsy.

Lewy Body Dementia: [25] Just like frontotemporal disease, identifying Lewy body dementia is also challenging as its symptoms might be confused with symptoms of other brain diseases. This disease also does not have a treatment and few medications and therapies may work for a time period but it cannot cure Lewy body dementia.

Parkinson's Disease: [26] Tests like single-photon emission computerized tomography (SPECT), called as dopamine transporter (DAT) scan is suggested. MRI and

PET scans can also be prescribed by some doctors. Carbidopa-levodopa (Rytary, Sinemet etc.,) are used as medicines in Parkinson's disease. Researches are trying to detect Parkinson's disease before the beginning of the symptoms. In a 2023 study, spinal fluid of more than 1,000 people were tested to look for clumps of alpha-synuclein protein. This protein is found is Lewy bodies and they form clumps which cannot be broken down by the body. Spreading of these clumps causes damages in the brain cells.

Multiple Sclerosis: [27] There is no particular test to diagnose multiple sclerosis. A number of tests like blood tests, spinal tap, MRI, evoked potential tests are recommended to diagnose multiple sclerosis. However, there is no treatment from multiple sclerosis. Corticosteroids like oral prednisone and intravenous methylprednisolone are prescribed. Early stages of multiple sclerosis can be treated by plasma exchange.

Amyotrophic Lateral Sclerosis: Just like multiple sclerosis, there is no particular test to diagnose amyotrophic lateral sclerosis. FDA approved medicine for ALS is riluzole. Using this drug has helped people diagnosed with ALS survive longer.

Progressive Supranuclear Palsy (PSP): This disease is often mistaken as Parkinson's disease and so, diagnosing this disease is not easy. There are no treatments and no way to slow down the effects of progressive supranuclear palsy. Frew treatments like oral medications, therapies, eye treatments can help to manage the symptoms of this disease better.

Creutzfeldt-Jakob Disease: [28] There is no effective treatment for any of the variants of Creutzfeldt-Jakob disease and as of now the medicines tested for this disease has not shown any benefits.

Huntington's Disease: [29] There is no effective treatment for Huntington's Disease. Diagnosis is done initially by a general physical exam and neurological and psychiatric examinations. Family medical history is also taken into consideration. The neurologist tests the patients motor, sensory and psychiatric symptoms. Just like in other neurodegenerative diseases, MRI and CT scans are recommended to patients based on their conditions. Standardized test to check memory, reasoning, emotional state, behavioral patterns etc., are conducted. If the symptoms match with those of Huntington's disease, then a genetic test is prescribed for the nontypical gene. Hence the disease is confirmed after diagnosis.

Medications can lessen the symptom of Huntington's disease. For movement disorders, drugs like tetrabenazine (Xena zine) and deutetrabenazine (Austedo), haloperidol and fluphenazine, olanzapine (Zyprexa) and aripiprazole (Abilify) are prescribed. Other medications like amantadine (Gocovri, Osmolex ER), levetiracetam (Keppra, Elepsia XR, Spritam) and clonazepam (Klonopin) may also help.

For psychiatric disorder, antidepressants like citalopram and fluoxetine, antipsychotic drugs like quetiapine and olanzapine, and mood-stabilizing drugs like divalproex and carbamazepine may be prescribed.

2 Ai in Neurodegenerative Diseases

[1] So far, we have seen how the neurodegenerative diseases are increasing in number day by day in the older population. We have also seen that neurodegenerative disease is not a specific type of disease. However, this term has a lot of different types of diseases within it as Alzheimer's disease, Parkinson's disease, frontotemporal disease, multiple sclerosis and others. These diseases are so dangerous and some of these diseases may even cause death in within 1–5 years of its outbreak. Looking at the diagnosis and treatment conditions for these diseases, it is evident that figuring out what type of the neurodegenerative disease is there is a very tedious task to do. Several tests, therapies and medicines can only lead us to just figure out what type of disease a patient is suffering through. Also, there is no proper medicine that will suit all the patients for a specific type of disease, and most importantly, there is no cure for neurodegenerative diseases. Diagnosing as we have understood is a long procedure that takes a really long time. The time during which a patient is being diagnosed can worsen up the situations. Hence several AI/ML models are being used to advance the technology and identify the type of neurodegenerative disease in lesser time.

2.1 Blood Transcript Biomarkers Identification by Machine Learning Algorithm

As we have seen, identification of certain biomarkers in the blood can help us identify if a patient is suffering through a neurodegenerative disease or not. The currents methods are highly expensive and time consuming. Using machine learning models can help us identify and distinguish neurodegenerative diseases like Alzheimer's disease, Parkinson's disease, amyotrophic lateral sclerosis, Friedreich's ataxia, Huntington's disease or frontotemporal disease in affected individuals from healthy individuals. All this can be done with lesser cost, in a faster manner, with minimal invasiveness and can be accessible by any medical clinic in the world. A small set of blood transcripts are taken from the patients. Using existing datasets of the patients, a machine learning model is being formed depending on the accuracy of the test results.

Several machine learning models, such as deep neural networks, random forests, and support vector machines are used to form several models in the medical field. Of these models, random forest and DNNs are used for identifying biomarkers as they give the best results compared to other machine learning models (Fig. 12).

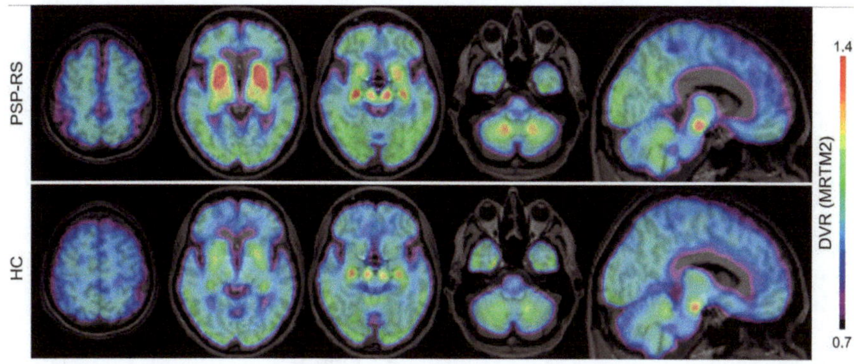

Fig. 12 Blood transcript biomarker identification through PET scan [18]

2.2 *Random Forest Model for Identifying Biomarkers*

What is Random Forest?

Random forest is a machine learning algorithm that is used for both classification and regression problems in ML. It belongs to the supervised learning technique and is based on the concept of ensemble learning. Ensemble learning is a process which combines multiple classifiers to solve a complex problem and improve performance of the model. So basically, the classifier random forest contains a number of decision trees on various subsets of the given dataset and it takes the average of the dataset to improve the accuracy of prediction.

[30, 31] Prediction from each tree is taken and based on the majority votes, the algorithm predicts the final output. The more the number of trees in a forest, the higher the accuracy predicted. This prevents the problem of overfitting (Fig. 13).

Random Forest algorithm follows the follows steps to predict the results:

1. Selects random x data points from the data set
2. Build decision trees based on the selected data points
3. Choosing how many trees we want to make by selecting a number N
4. Repeating the steps 1 and 2.
5. Whenever a new data point is encountered, predictions for each decision tree is considered and the new data set is assigned to the one that wins with the majority votes.

2.3 *Random Forest Feature Selection Methods*

[32] Boruta, permutation-based feature selection, permutation-based feature selection with correction, and backward elimination-based feature selection methods are the four methods that were applied to automatically select important features.

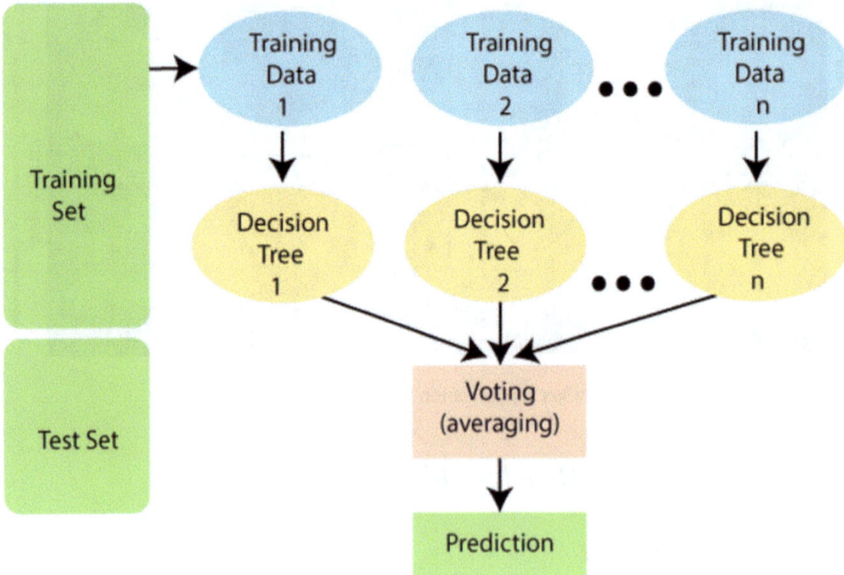

Fig. 13 How random forest algorithm works? [21]

Boruta

Permutation-Based Feature Selection

Recursive Feature Elimination

2.3.1 Artificial Intelligence for Alzheimer' Disease

[24, 33] In Alzheimer's disease, amyloid plaques and neurofibrillary tangles are the neuropathological hallmarks. These can be evaluated with the help of neuroimaging and cerebrospinal fluid (CSF) biomarker assessment. The ratio of amyloidβ1-42 (Aβ42) with amyloid β1-40 (Aβ42/Aβ40), total tau protein (t-tau), and hyperphosphorylated tau (p-tau181) is considered. Years of clinical research has led us to discover several ways of pathogenesis, but the etiology of AD is still misunderstood. All the data from electronic health records and multi-omics sciences has given us with unlimited amount of information about biological processes, such as genomes, transcriptomes, and proteomes. All of these can be explored through Big Data exploitation.

[30] Complex AI-based models can extract successful and meaningful information from big data, but as the complexity increases, interpreting how the model is producing results more and more complex. The major problem of AI technology is to

make AI explainable to patients and clinicians, as they need to trust with the research to believe the health predictions made by AI. In order to efficiently use the biological experiments, complex biological modeling is required, which is based on mathematical and statistical tools, such as Artificial Neural Networks. AI can use the features of Machine Learning (ML) and Deep Learning (DL) to develop algorithms that can help us classify the patient based on the processing of a large amount of data like data sources, neuroimaging, biochemical markers, clinical, and neuropsychological (NPS) data (Fig. 14).

Random Forest Algorithm is used for statistical analysis and the datasets are trained based on various conditions to predict the outcome (Fig. 15).

[34] AI techniques are widely being used to get faster and automated results, and the accuracy of the early prediction is also increasing. The algorithm is trained to get the early predictions. The regression task predicts the value of a variable which is measured on a continuous scale. AI pipelines can be applied in automatic compound synthesis. After cell or organoid-based experiments, the AI model can be updated by which AI can propose a new molecular optimization plan and the conduction of new bioassays. This can help with the automated drug development cycle. This has so much impact on the medical world as it can help with the invention of new drugs for Alzheimer's disease. Using AI algorithms, the participant selection can be optimized as some patients may not respond to the drugs predicted, or may have drug reaction due to their sensitivity to that drug.

Can AI Predict AD Early?

Well, the topic is very interesting. So far, we have seen that machine learning and deep learning models have used publicly available datasets and biobanks to predict outcome for a patient based on certain factors. Tests like Magnetic Resonance Imaging (MRI), Positron Emission Tomography (PET) and other tests have given detailed description about a patient's conditions which has added a lot of value in the prediction of the disease. Using this information, the model is trained every time with more and more generated data. ML is used in the CAD of many pathologies, of which Alzheimer's is one of the most important (Fig. 16).

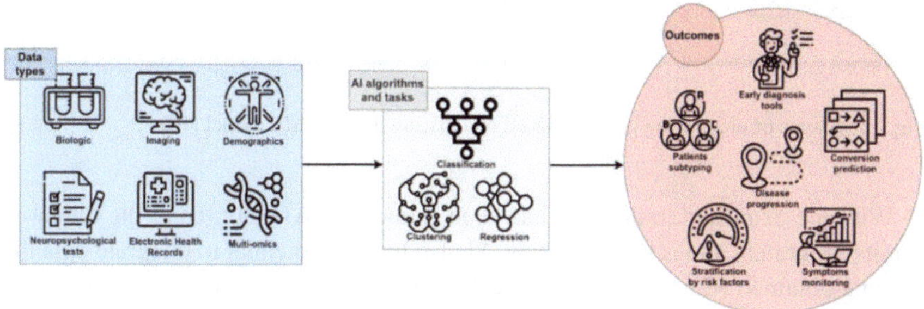

Fig. 14 AI algorithms taking existing data sets and computing outcomes [20]

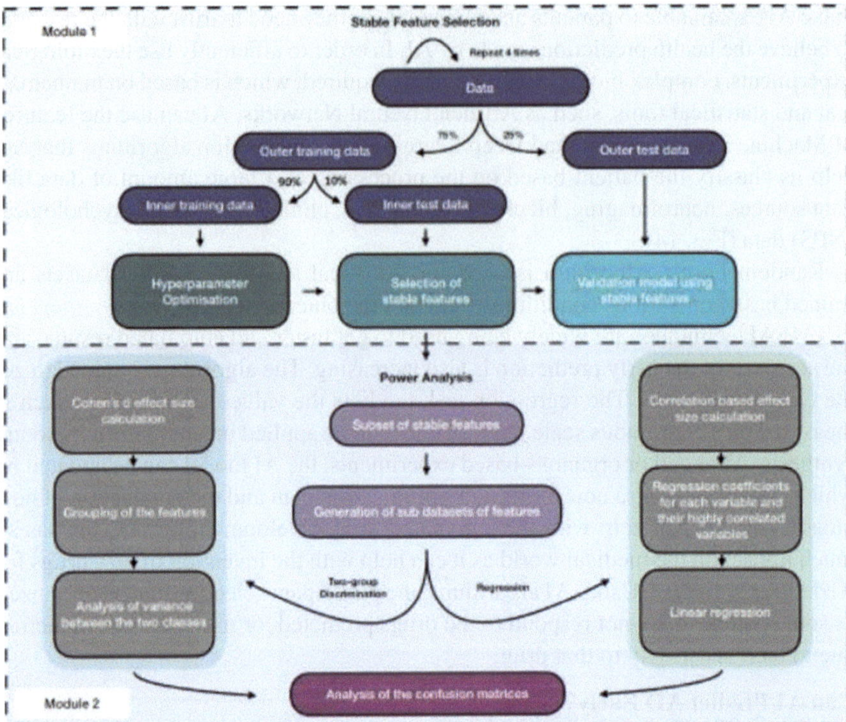

Fig. 15 AI models selecting features and calculating several results [24]

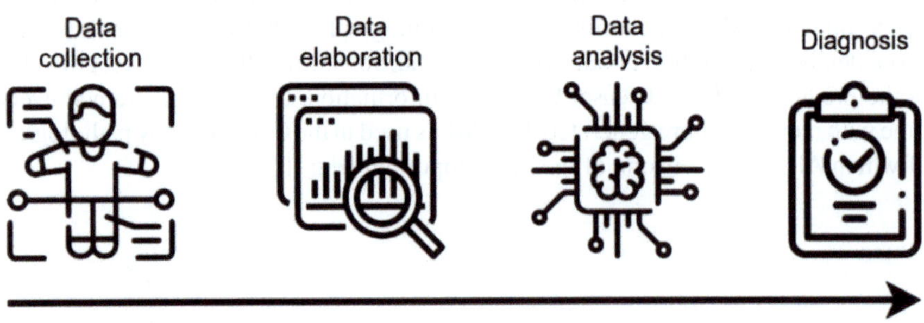

Fig. 16 Stages of diagnosing patients based on existing data By ML model [10]

With the extensive training, it has been found that AI can predict the diagnosis results accurately and is being trusted. AI also has the potential to integrate data that is being obtained with the use of new technologies. These may include, devices used for evaluation of language and verbal fluency in the patients. Using all these types of integration and prediction, we can say that AI can predict AD early. However, more research and study is still on ongoing matter to improve the efficiency of AI technologies so that it can be used with more reliability.

Prediction of MCI to AD Conversion:

[35] Mild Cognitive Impairment (MCI) is the early symptoms or neurodegenerative diseases that. These impairments are usually reversible if caught at a very early stage. Else the symptoms keep on growing over time. Diagnosing and detecting these symptoms at an early stage is really important so minimize the effects with proper medications. AI can easily classify the symptoms with high accuracy with the help of the available datasets and neuroimaging data. Several predictive models have been developed, which gives highest accuracy values (100%) in AD vs. NC classification. But AI models can give results with so much accuracy when the patient is suffering from moderate-severe Alzheimer's. Detecting and diagnosing the symptoms during early stage is difficult even for AI models as the early-stage symptoms for Alzheimer's overlaps with those of Parkinson's and other neurodegenerative diseases.

The algorithms are divided into two parts to distinguish between two groups of people to predict MCI to AD conversion:

1. Patients who will convert from MCI to AD in a given time period (usually 3 years)
2. Patients who will not convert from MCI to AD

[32] Dividing the two types of people makes it a little bit easier to diagnose the patients individually. It is estimated that each year nearly 15% of patients convert from MCI to AD.

An ensemble model is developed by training different supervised ML models based on the ADNI data set, socio-demographic characteristics, clinical scale ratings, and NPS test scores. This model gives a highly accurate performance which an AUC of 0.88 in predicting the conversion. This model uses only non-invasive and easily collectable predictors which increases its potential.

A DL model was trained using the same data sets to predict MCI to AD as well as AD vs. NC classification. All the data was processed in a multi-modal feature extraction phase in order to combine all the data together and get a classification output. The model predicted nearly 100% accurate results for AD vs. NC classification, and 0.925 AUC with 86% accuracy for MCI to AD transformation prediction.

MRI and PET data are independently modeled by ML algorithms for CAD systems which yields a good accuracy for prediction. Integrating neuroimaging data with variables like, cognitive measures, biochemical changes etc., can drastically improve the performance of the model. We can also call it as integrating multi-modal data.

Analyzing all of the models developed through different types of data sets training gave us efficient models to accurately detect the type of biomarkers and give high predictivity in both plasma and CSF which helped with making plasma a alternative for CSF (Fig. 17).

AI in Predicting the Course and Progression of Alzheimer's Disease:

[35] The rate at which the disease is spreading in a patient's body is important to monitor to properly diagnose and prescribe the patient with suitable drugs. As

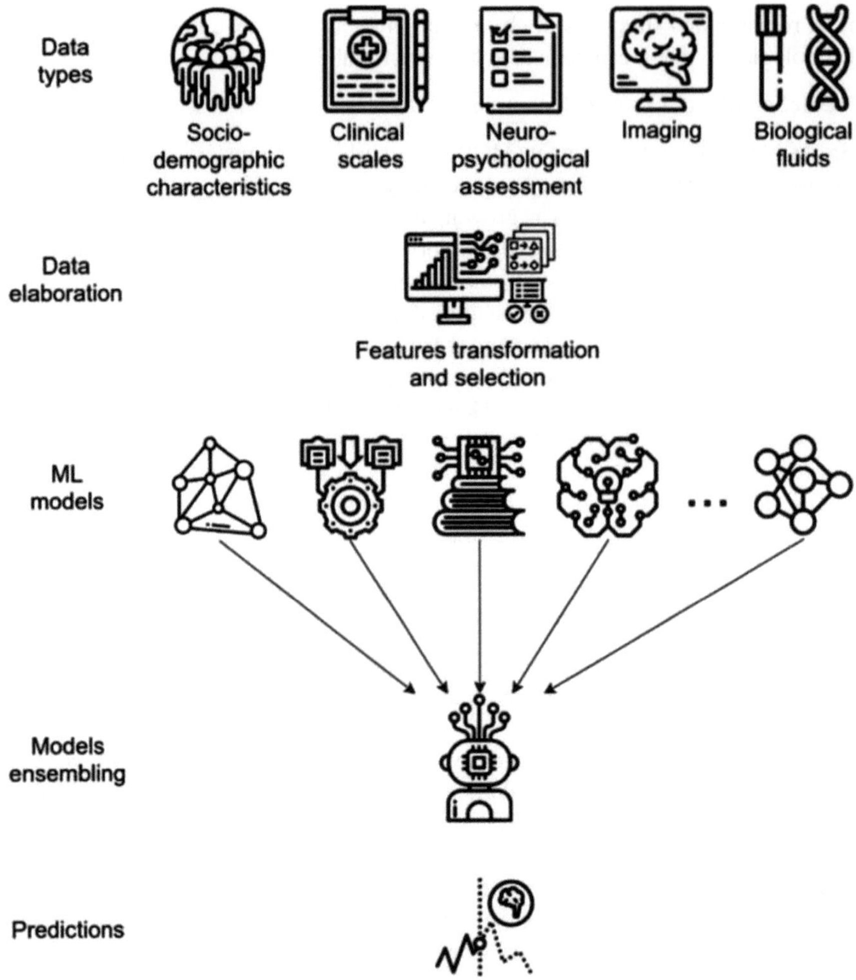

Fig. 17 Ensemble-based model predicting the transformation of mci patients to ad patients with classification [25]

discussed in the previous section, the model trained on NPS test scores and other data sets are used to predict the disease. According to research, transcranial magnetic stimulation evaluates alteration of mechanisms of cortical plasticity in order to predict clinical progression to dementia. Prodromal AD and MCI patients who convert to AD patients within 3 years have impaired Long-Term Potentiation (LTP) significantly compared to patients who don't convert from MCI to AD. This information helps in the ADNI database which offers multi-modal data. Models fit better when trained over multi-modal data with cognitive data and biological data.

Multi-modal neuroimaging and clinical data can be used to estimate the time conversion from [36, 37] MCI patients to AD patients, even when the data is incomplete or noisy. Regression model with ADNI multi-modal data is made to find the risk factors in conversion from MCI to AD. Autosomal-dominant AD data (which includes amyloid-PET, FDG-PET, structural MRI, and CSF) were used to derive a prognostic index from increasingly complex biomarker data. The model showed to have accuracy in predicting the cognitive decline in AD patients.

Hence, we can conclude that AI model is helpful in predicting the course and progression of Alzheimer's disease.

2.4 Conclusion

[35] We can conclude that with the help of AI and several Machine Learning, Deep Learning and Transfer Learning techniques, many models can be made which can help in the identification of the disease, prediction of MCI to AD conversion rate, and prediction of course and progression of the disease. So, we can say that AI is helping medical science with dealing neurodegenerative diseases in an efficient, cost-effective, faster and minimum invasive manner. Random forest classification and ensemble-based learning has proven to give the most accurate results in detecting and diagnosing the disease. With time, AI is proving to increase its efficiency in predicting the results.

2.5 Challenges for AI in Neurodegenerative Diseases

From the applications of AI in Alzheimer's Disease, we can see that even though several models have been built up to easily and effectively calculate the predictions for biomarkers and diagnose the disease, it is still hard for AI to predict the results without any problems. AI may have proven to give accurate results in a cost-effective and faster manner, but there is no particular model used in the medical field to diagnose a patient. This is because which model gives accuracy at which time is unpredictable. Also, existing data sets can only help with the classification of disease to a certain extent but AI stills lacks to predict the type of neurodegenerative disease a patient is suffering from because of the similarities in the symptoms of the diseases. This might lead to the ML model to predict the disease incorrectly. Also, there are variations in the biomarkers found in patients which increases the complexity to understand which type of biomarker is present in the brain cells of the patient. If the biomarker is not identified correctly, then it cannot be predicted why the nerve cells are deteriorating and what type of protein is being accumulated which may lead to the deterioration of the nerve cells. AI is just a growing concept and with limiting knowledge about the data sets and difficulty in predicting early-stage disease symptoms, it becomes even more challenging to prescribe a patient with a particular type of drug. As we have seen that there is no cure for neurodegenerative diseases, and there is no single drug that can suit all the patients with the same type of disease [38–40]. It becomes more challenging for Artificial Intelligence based models to predict the drugs that will suit a patient. AI based model screenings are done individually for each patient to understand what will suit the patient which can slow down the diagnosing process. In many cases, a drug which doesn't suit a patient can instead lead to the growth of the disease in the body and can cause several side-affects. Hence, a model which can predict the drug course for a patient accurately is a bug challenge. Also, to predict the progression of disease inside a patient's body, it is required that the model used is highly predictive. So, even though AI is a fast-progressing technology, it still needs improvement in certain areas to fully start functioning in the medical field.

2.6 Opportunities for AI in Neurodegenerative Diseases

Although there are certain drawbacks of using AI in the field of neurodegenerative diseases, it is worthy to note that the technology has led to a lot of advancement in this field. With the help of ML and DL based models, identification of biomarkers has become faster. Although a lot of training is required, the models can predict the diseases and through individual screening, AI can accurately predict the progression of diseases and prescribe drugs. Using AI is reducing the cost that is spent on several tests like MRI, CT scan, PET, neuroimaging etc., which are very costly. Multiple methods of diagnosing with therapies included has made it even more time-consuming with high invasiveness to diagnose the patient. Using AI has definitely reduced the time taken to diagnose the patients and with minimal invasiveness.

Advancement in AI can help with the development of models that can be permanently used in the field of medical sciences. Till now there is no cure for neurodegenerative diseases but as AI is rapidly progressing, we can expect that Artificial Intelligence applications can help us find proper diagnosing methods and find a cure for the respective diseases. Although, identification of the diseases at the early onset might be challenging, but with the help of increasing data sets along with tests results and neuroimaging, it would be possible for AI based models to predict the diseases during its onset and predict the diseases accurately. In a very less time, AI has shown tremendous support in this field and has shown to be reliable for accurately predicting the results. As the models keep on training, the efficiency of the model is increased and we can expect that sooner, AI based models can be officially used in diagnosing the patients with neurodegenerative diseases. AI has made it easier to classify the type of disease a patient is suffering from [41–45]. However, to gain confidence of the patients as well as the medical people (doctors, testing units) in AI, it would be crucial for the models to grow in terms of accuracy and speed.

Definitely, AI has helped the researchers to give a solution in making the diagnosing process a lot easier. There is still a lot of work to be done to finally depend on AI for diagnosing the diseases. AI has a lot of potential and it can impact the lives of people suffering from neurodegenerative diseases in a positive way. It has a lot of scope and studying about it is an on-going process to come up with a solution that will help medical science in terms of efficiency and accuracy, and the patients in terms of money and trust.

3 Conclusion

Neurogenerative diseases is a huge challenge in human beings especially in the Elderly people especially above the age of 65. The diseases include Alzheimer's disease, Parkinson's disease, Lewy body dementia, frontotemporal disease, multiple sclerosis, amyotrophic lateral sclerosis, Huntington's disease, Chromatic Traumatic Encephalopathy, progressive supranuclear palsy. All the above diseases permanently incurable and diagnosing these diseases is very expensive and drugs for no two patients may not be same. Therefore, many of researchers are trying to identify ways to diagnose these cases by using artificial Intelligence which helps to predict symptoms and classify the patients with various symptoms and developing a customized drug recommendation system using various techniques. In this chapter, we reviewed various neurogenerative diseases and their symptoms. We have also studied various AI techniques to diagnose neurogenerative diseases in a detailed manner.

References

1. Tăuţan, A.-M., Ionescu, B., & Santarnecchi, E. (2021). Artificial intelligence in neurodegenerative diseases: A review of available tools with a focus on machine learning techniques. *Artificial Intelligence in Medicine, 117*, 102081.
2. Armstrong, R. (2020). What causes neurodegenerative disease? *Folia Neuropathologica, 58*(2), 93–112.
3. Uchida, A. et al. (2020). Correlation between brain volume and retinal photoreceptor outer segment volume in normal aging and neurodegenerative diseases. *PloS One, 15*(9), e0237078.
4. Richards, M., & Brayne, C. (2010). What do we mean by Alzheimer's disease? *BMJ*, 341.
5. Taplo, Y. M., Madianung, A., & Kanine, E. (2019). Aktivitas Bermain Domino Sebagai Media Untuk Meningkatkan Kemampuan Fungsi Kognitif Berhitung Pada Lansia. *Jurnal Keperawatan, 7*(1).
6. Bang, J., Spina, S., & Miller, B. L. (2015). Frontotemporal dementia. *The Lancet, 386*(10004), 1672–1682.
7. Kurz, A. et al. (2019). What is frontotemporal dementia?. *Maturitas, 79*(2), 216–219.
8. Thakur, S. P. et al. (2019). Skull-stripping of glioblastoma MRI scans using 3D deep learning. *International MICCAI Brainlesion Workshop*. Cham: Springer International Publishing.
9. McKee, A. C. et al. (2015). The neuropathology of chronic traumatic encephalopathy. *Brain Pathology, 25*(3), 350–364.
10. Turner, R. C. et al. (2013). Repetitive traumatic brain injury and development of chronic traumatic encephalopathy: a potential role for biomarkers in diagnosis, prognosis, and treatment?. *Frontiers in Neurology, 3*, 186.
11. Taylor, C. A., Bouldin, E. D., & McGuire, L. C. (2018). Subjective cognitive decline among adults aged $\geq$ 45 years—United States, 2015–2016. *Morbidity and Mortality Weekly Report, 67*(27), 753.

12. Fell, K., & Gupta, J. (2023). Lewy body dementia. *Primary Care Occupational Therapy: A Quick Reference Guide*. Cham: Springer Nature Switzerland, 163–171.
13. Daugherty, J., & Sarmiento, K. (2018). Chronic traumatic encephalopathy: What do parents of youth athletes know about it? *Brain injury, 32*(13–14), 1773–1779.
14. Dobson, R., & Giovannoni, G. (2019). Multiple sclerosis–a review. *European Journal of Neurology, 26*(1), 27–40.
15. Kiernan, M. C. et al. (2011). Amyotrophic lateral sclerosis. *The Lancet, 377*(9769), 942–955.
16. Martin, S., Al Khleifat, A., & Al-Chalabi, A. (2017). What causes amyotrophic lateral sclerosis? *F1000Research*, 6.
17. Ikram, S. et al. (2021). Progressive supranuclear palsy: A case report and literature review. *Archives of Clinical and Medical Case Reports, 5*(6), 838–845.
18. Höglinger, G. U. et al. (2011). Identification of common variants influencing risk of the tauopathy progressive supranuclear palsy. *Nature Genetics, 43*(7), 699–705.
19. Atkinson, A., Mary, J., & Sonja Carol Orff. (2019). Prions to Pathways: Safeguarding Against Creutzfeldt-Jakob Disease in the Operating Room.
20. Prusiner, S. B. (2001). Neurodegenerative diseases and prions. *New England Journal of Medicine, 344*(20), 1516–1526.
21. Petersen, R. C. (2016). Mild cognitive impairment. *CONTINUUM: Lifelong Learning in Neurology* 22.2 Dementia, 404.
22. Durães, F., Pinto, M., & Sousa, E. (2018). Old drugs as new treatments for neurodegenerative diseases. *Pharmaceuticals, 11*(2), 44.
23. Valenza, M., & Scuderi, C. (2022). How useful are biomarkers for the diagnosis of Alzheimer's disease and especially for its therapy? *Neural Regeneration Research, 17*(10), 2205.
24. Sperling, R. et al. (2012). Amyloid-related imaging abnormalities in patients with Alzheimer's disease treated with bapineuzumab: A retrospective analysis. *The Lancet Neurology, 11*(3), 241–249.
25. Hanson, J. C., & Lippa, C. F. (2009). Lewy body dementia. *International Review of Neurobiology, 84*, 215–228.
26. Jankovic, J., & Giselle Aguilar, L. (2008). Current approaches to the treatment of Parkinson's disease. *Neuropsychiatric Disease and Treatment, 4*(4), 743–757.
27. Goldenberg, M. M. (2012). Multiple sclerosis review. *Pharmacy and Therapeutics, 37*(3), 175.
28. Centers for Disease Control and Prevention. (2017). Creutzfeldt-Jakob disease, classic (CJD). *Im Internet: http://www.cdc.gov/prions/cjd/index. html (Stand: 10.08. 2018).*
29. Frank, S. (2014). Treatment of Huntington's disease. *Neurotherapeutics, 11*, 153–160.
30. Huseby, C. J. et al. (2022). Blood transcript biomarkers selected by machine learning algorithm classify neurodegenerative diseases including Alzheimer's disease. *Biomolecules, 12*(11), 1592.
31. Acharjee, A. et al. (2020). A random forest based biomarker discovery and power analysis framework for diagnostics research. *BMC Medical Genomics, 13*(1), 1–14.
32. Charbuty, B., & Abdulazeez, A. (2021). Classification based on decision tree algorithm for machine learning. *Journal of Applied Science and Technology Trends, 2*(01), 20–28.
33. Martinez, B., & Peplow, P. V. (2022). MicroRNA biomarkers in frontotemporal dementia and to distinguish from Alzheimer's disease and amyotrophic lateral sclerosis. *Neural Regeneration Research, 17*(7), 1412.
34. Zhang, J. et al. (2023). Machine learning on visibility graph features discriminates the cognitive event-related potentials of patients with early Alzheimer's disease from healthy aging. *Brain Sciences, 13*(5), 770.
35. Fabrizio, C. et al. (2021). Artificial intelligence for Alzheimer's disease: promise or challenge?. *Diagnostics, 11*(8), 1473.
36. Giannone, M. et al. (2021). Seeing Beyond: OT's role in low vision in individuals with neurodegenerative disease.
37. Marsden, C. D. (1994). Parkinson's disease. *Journal of Neurology, Neurosurgery, and Psychiatry, 57*(6), 672.

38. https://tse4.mm.bing.net/th?id=OIP.DEPq0rziwDM9SZ_UXWY1NQHaF-&pid=Api&P=0&h=180
39. https://www.frontiersin.org/files/Articles/691136/fncel-15-691136-HTML/image_m/fncel-15-691136-g001.jpg
40. https://www.mkexpress.net/wpcontent/uploads/2021/04/amyotrophic-lateral-sclerosis.jpg
41. http://s3.amazonaws.com/rdcmssnmmi/files/production/public/docs/pr/SNMMI2019_Brendel_Supranuclear-Palsy_Figure.jpg
42. https://www.ncbi.nlm.nih.gov/core/lw/2.0/html/tileshop_pmc/tileshop_pmc_inline.html?title=Click%20on%20image%20to%20zoom&p=PMC3&id=8391160_diagnostics-11-01473-g001.jpg
43. https://www.ncbi.nlm.nih.gov/core/lw/2.0/html/tileshop_pmc/tileshop_pmc_inline.html?title=Click%20on%20image%20to%20zoom&p=PMC3&id=7685541_12920_2020_826_Fig1_HTML.jpg
44. https://www.ncbi.nlm.nih.gov/core/lw/2.0/html/tileshop_pmc/tileshop_pmc_inline.html?title=Click%20on%20image%20to%20zoom&p=PMC3&id=8391160_diagnostics-11-01473-g002.jpg
45. https://www.ncbi.nlm.nih.gov/core/lw/2.0/html/tileshop_pmc/tileshop_pmc_inline.html?title=Click%20on%20image%20to%20zoom&p=PMC3&id=8391160_diagnostics-11-01473-g003.jpg

Artificial Intelligence in Neuro Degenerative Diseases: Opportunities and Challenges

Sivaramakrishnan Rajaraman

Abstract This chapter delves into the transformative role of Artificial Intelligence (AI) in understanding, detecting, and treating neurodegenerative diseases, a subject of great relevance given the global rise of these complex disorders. AI's role in medical diagnosis forms the crux of the initial discussion, setting the stage for a detailed examination of AI techniques tailored for neurodegenerative diseases. We then explore the multifaceted applications of AI, encompassing disease detection, diagnosis, progression modeling, and personalized treatment recommendations, with emphasis on their strengths and potential limitations. The case studies provide practical insights into the deployment of AI in real-world clinical settings. Subsequently, we discuss vital challenges confronting the integration of AI in neurodegenerative disease detection, including data privacy, AI model interpretability, potential biases, technological and resource constraints, as well as ethical and regulatory considerations. Shifting the focus to the future, we envisage opportunities poised at the intersection of AI and neurodegenerative diseases. These include AI-enabled drug discovery and the role of AI in advancing neuroimaging techniques, both of which promise a paradigm shift in our approach to managing these diseases. In conclusion, we encapsulate the key takeaways and potential future directions. By exploring AI's myriad possibilities, this chapter underscores the potential of these technologies in revolutionizing neurodegenerative disease detection and management while also grappling with the challenges that accompany this new frontier in healthcare.

Keywords Artificial intelligence · Neurodegenerative diseases · Disease detection and diagnosis · AI-Enabled drug discovery · Advancements in neuroimaging

S. Rajaraman (✉)
International Drive, Guidehouse Inc, McLean, VA 22102, USA
e-mail: sivaramakrishnan.rajaraman@guidehouse.com

© The Author(s), under exclusive license to Springer Nature Switzerland AG 2024

L. Gaur et al. (eds.), *AI and Neuro-Degenerative Diseases*, Studies in Computational Intelligence 1131, https://doi.org/10.1007/978-3-031-53148-4_8

1 Introduction

Artificial intelligence (AI), differing from natural human or animal intelligence, signifies machine intelligence that encompasses capabilities such as language translation, speech recognition, computer vision, and automated decision-making [1]. AI, established as an academic discipline in 1956, is paving the way for the current prevalence of statistical machine learning (ML) techniques. Neurodegenerative diseases are a major category of disorders impacting the central and peripheral nervous systems, hallmarked by the progressive degeneration of neurons leading to their death [2]. Examples include Alzheimer's disease, Parkinson's disease, Huntington's disease, amyotrophic lateral sclerosis (ALS), and others. These diseases remain incurable, warranting extensive research into their multi-faceted aspects. Neurons form the complex biological wiring that facilitates cognition, memory, movement, sensation, and emotion. Their loss disrupts neural networks, leading to cognitive deficits, movement disorders, and uncontrolled muscle activity [3]. Common across all neurodegenerative diseases is the accumulation of misfolded proteins, causing neuronal dysfunction and death. For instance, Alzheimer's disease is associated with beta-amyloid plaques and neurofibrillary tangles, while Parkinson's disease is characterized by alpha-synuclein aggregates, known as Lewy bodies [4]. Oxidative stress and inflammation have also been studied for their roles in neurodegenerative diseases [5]. Treatments using antioxidants and anti-inflammatory drugs have been explored for their potential utility in managing these diseases, though they cannot halt or reverse neuronal degeneration. One promising avenue of research involves repurposing drugs by identifying shared pathophysiological features between different neurodegenerative diseases, which could expedite the drug development process [6].

2 Role of AI in Medical Diagnosis

The inception of AI in medical diagnosis can be traced back to the mid-twentieth century with early systems such as Dendral and MYCIN, developed in the 1960s and 70s respectively, leveraging AI principles to assist in medical diagnosis [7, 8]. Later in the 1980s and 90s, further progress was made with the creation of expert systems like CASNET, INTERNIST-I, and QMR that harnessed complex rule-based algorithms, expanding AI's role in medicine and proposing automation potential [9, 10].

Despite these advancements, the inability of rule-based systems to manage large data volumes and the requirement for substantial manual intervention led to the advent of ML systems in the late twentieth century. ML algorithms significantly enhanced AI capabilities and led to widespread usage in medical diagnosis, particularly in areas like image-based diagnosis, genomics, and personalized medicine [11].

Presently, AI's role in healthcare is multifaceted, greatly influencing image-based and data-driven diagnoses. In image-based diagnosis, deep learning (DL) techniques such as convolutional neural networks (CNNs) have shown promise in interpreting medical images, aiding in early disease detection [12]. This can be seen in tools like Google's DeepMind and IBM's Watson Health, used for interpreting radiological images and pathology slides. Concurrently, data-driven diagnosis employs AI for structured and unstructured data analysis from electronic health records (EHRs) and genomics, thus aiding in disease detection and prognosis prediction, especially in the field of precision medicine [13, 14].

The integration of AI with the Internet of Things (IoT) has resulted in the emergence of wearable health technologies that provide continuous health monitoring and early disease detection [15, 16]. However, concerns regarding the black-box nature of AI models, data privacy, and the requirement for robust validation and regulation are continually influencing the evolving landscape of AI in medical diagnosis [17].

3 AI Techniques for Neurodegenerative Diseases

3.1 Supervised Learning Algorithms

Supervised learning algorithms operate based on labeled input–output pairs [18]. The algorithm learns to predict the output from the input data during the training phase, and this learned knowledge is then used to make predictions on new, unseen data. One of the most widely used supervised learning algorithms is logistic regression [19]. The logistic regression model predicts the probability that a given input point belongs to a certain category. Mathematically, the model predicts *y (output)* from *x (input)* as:

$$y = 1/(1 + exp(-(b0 + b1 * x))) \tag{1}$$

Here, *exp* denotes the exponential function, *b0* is the y-intercept, and *b1* is the slope. In the context of neurodegenerative diseases, logistic regression can be used to predict the probability of a patient having a specific disease based on various predictors like age, family history, genetic factors, and more [20].

Another prominent supervised learning algorithm is the support vector machine (SVM) [21], which works well with high-dimensional data, making it suitable for neuroimaging data. SVM constructs a hyperplane in a high-dimensional space that maximally separates the classes. If y is the output and x is the input, the decision function for SVM is given by,

$$y = sign(w^T x + b) \tag{2}$$

Here, w is the weight vector, T is the transpose, and b is the bias. The features extracted from clinical data and brain volumes can be fed into the SVMs that serve as classifiers for classifying various neurodegenerative diseases such as Alzheimer's disease [22].

3.2 Unsupervised Learning Algorithms

Unlike supervised learning, unsupervised learning algorithms operate on unlabeled data [23]. The aim is to find underlying patterns or structures in the data. One of the widely used unsupervised learning algorithms is k-means clustering. It groups the data into k clusters such that the sum of squares from points to the assigned cluster centers is minimized. The objective function J for k-means is given by,

$$J = \Sigma\Sigma||x(i) - \mu(j)||^2 \quad (3)$$

Here, the value of i ranges over all points, j ranges over all clusters, $x(i)$ are the data points, and $\mu(j)$ are the cluster centers. In neurodegenerative diseases, unsupervised learning can be used to identify subgroups of patients with similar characteristics, which could help in understanding disease heterogeneity and tailoring treatment strategies [24].

3.3 Reinforcement Learning Algorithms

Reinforcement learning (RL) is a type of ML where an agent learns to make decisions by interacting with its environment. The agent performs certain actions and gets rewards or penalties. Over time, it learns the best strategy, called policy, to get the maximum reward [25]. Q-learning, a model-free RL algorithm, can be used for finding an optimal policy [25]. If s is the current state, a is the action, r is the reward, and α is the learning rate, the Q value is updated as,

$$Q(s, a) \leftarrow Q(s, a) + \alpha[r + \gamma max Q(s\prime, a\prime) - Q(s, a)] \quad (4)$$

Here, γ is the discount factor, and s' and a' are the next state and action, respectively. In neurodegenerative diseases, RL can be used in personalized treatment strategies, where the algorithm can learn the optimal treatment policy for a patient based on the patient's responses to previous treatments [26].

3.4 DL Algorithms

DL models, a subset of ML, have transformed the field of AI and are increasingly being employed in neurodegenerative disease research due to their ability to automatically learn and improve from experience without being explicitly programmed [27]. This is especially true with large, high-dimensional, and complex neuroimaging datasets. Different types of DL models have been employed, including CNNs, Recurrent Neural Networks (RNNs), and Long Short-Term Memory (LSTM) networks. CNNs, inspired by the organization of the animal visual cortex, have been extensively applied to neuroimaging data due to their high performance in image analysis tasks. CNNs have been applied to classify Alzheimer's disease and mild cognitive impairment from neuroimaging data, outperforming traditional machine learning approaches [26, 27].

RNNs are another class of neural networks that are particularly useful when dealing with sequential data, which arises naturally in the study of neurodegenerative diseases where patient data are collected over time [28]. The hidden state in a recurrent neuron at time *t*, *h(t)*, is a function of the input at that time *x(t)*, and the hidden state of the previous time step *h(t-1)*. In the simple case of a vanilla RNN, this function is given as,

$$h(t) = f(Wxh * x(t) + Whh * h(t-1) + bh) \tag{5}$$

Here, *Wxh*, *Whh*, and *bh* are the parameters of the model, and *f* is a non-linear function like *tanh*. However, vanilla RNNs are difficult to train due to problems like exploding and vanishing gradients. Hence, a variant of RNN, the Long Short-Term Memory (LSTM) network, is more commonly used in practice [29]. LSTMs have a similar structure as a regular RNN but have a different function for computing the hidden state. This function includes mechanisms called gates that control the flow of information into and out of the memory cell, *c(t)*, given by,

$$f(t) = \sigma(Wf * [h(t-1), x(t)] + bf)$$

$$i(t) = \sigma(Wi * [h(t-1), x(t)] + bi)$$

$$o(t) = \sigma(Wo * [h(t-1), x(t)] + bo)$$

$$c(t) = f(t) * c(t-1) + i(t) * tanh(Wc * [h(t-1), x(t)] + bc)$$

$$h(t) = o(t) * tanh(c(t)) \tag{6}$$

Here, *f(t)*, *i(t)*, and *o(t)* are the forget, input, and output gates, respectively, σ is the sigmoid function, and the rest of the notation is the same as in the RNN equation. One successful application of LSTM is to model the progression of neurodegenerative diseases over time and predict future patient status [30].

DL models are also often combined in practice. For example, CNN-LSTM models combine CNN layers for feature extraction and LSTM layers for sequence prediction, taking advantage of both spatial and temporal modeling capabilities [31]. They have been used to analyze spatiotemporal neuroimaging data (like fMRI), where both spatial patterns and temporal sequences are important.

4 Applications of AI in Neurodegenerative Diseases

4.1 Disease Detection and Diagnosis

AI has revolutionized the detection and diagnosis of neurodegenerative diseases. Conventional ML/DL algorithms are used to analyze a myriad of data types such as neuroimaging data (MRI, PET, etc.), genetic data, cognitive tests, and more to predict the onset and diagnosis of diseases like Alzheimer's disease (AD), Parkinson's disease (PD), and Amyotrophic Lateral Sclerosis (ALS). One example is the use of CNNs for the analysis of neuroimaging data to detect AD. The study by [32] used CNNs for the classification of Alzheimer's disease using fMRI data. The model was trained to distinguish between different stages of Alzheimer's—Normal, Mild Cognitive Impairment (MCI), and severe AD, demonstrating high accuracy in its results. Similarly, acoustic signals were analyzed using a hybrid system for the diagnosis of PD [33]. The approach used linear discriminant analysis (LDA) to reduce the dimensionality of the voice signals and the model hyper-parameter optimization was performed using a genetic algorithm (GA).

4.2 Disease Progression Modeling

AI techniques also play a significant role in modeling the progression of neurodegenerative diseases. They are capable of predicting future disease status, and cognitive decline rate, and helping in prognosis determination. The study by [30] utilized longitudinal and multimodal biomarkers for predicting future clinical changes in MCI patients. The study proposed prognosticating forthcoming alterations in the clinical state of MCI patients utilizing both initial and progressive multimodal data. The process begins with the formation of a longitudinal feature selection procedure, purposely selecting cerebral regions across diverse moments in time for each modality. A sparse linear regression model is trained at each time point using imaging data and matching clinical scores, incorporating 'group regularization' to amalgamate weights pertinent to identify brain regions at various time points, thereby permitting the selection of brain regions contingent on the cumulative strength of multiple time points. Consequently, longitudinal characteristics from the original baseline and progressive data were extracted to more accurately represent changes in the selected brain regions. Finally, a multi-kernel SVM was employed to predict the features extracted from the chosen brain regions across different modalities. The validation of the proposed method was performed on 88 ADNI MCI subjects possessing MRI and FDG-PET data along with their corresponding clinical scores (MMSE and ADAS-Cog) at five distinct time points. The outcomes from all tests demonstrated that the proposed methodology outperformed traditional methods in the prediction of future clinical alterations in MCI patients.

4.3 Personalized Treatment Recommendations

AI provides a platform for personalized medicine in neurodegenerative diseases, facilitating tailored treatment plans for individual patients. By integrating genetic data, patient history, lifestyle factors, and more, AI models can generate personalized treatment strategies. A study by [34] developed software to generate personalized treatment recommendations through a precision-medicine approach targeting AD's biological drivers. Inputs related to AD included genomic data, biospecimen measurements, imaging data, medical histories, medications, allergies, comorbidities, relevant lifestyle factors, and neuropsychological testing results. The algorithm ranked the most likely disease-contributing physiological and lifestyle states, which were then incorporated into a personalized care plan delivered to physicians, with health coaches assisting to improve adherence. The sample group consisted of 40 individuals with Subjective Cognitive Decline (SCD) and Mild Cognitive Impairment (MCI). Post software analysis, all participants adhered to their treatment plans for an average duration of 8.4 months. Most subjects (80%) exhibited stable or improved memory function, as gauged by standardized cognitive evaluations. Cognitive assessments revealed substantial improvement within the SCD group and in the CNS-VS Executive domain in the combined group. Blood panel biomarker improvements were also observed over time. Although the overall improvement in selected biomarkers wasn't statistically significant, homocysteine levels showed a significant decrease. The study suggested that modifiable interlocking feedback loops constitute AD risk factors, highlighting the importance of personalized, multimodal treatments. The AI model took into account the patient's genetic profile, biomarker readings, and clinical history to suggest personalized drug combinations.

4.4 Case Studies

Case studies provide practical examples of AI implementation in neurodegenerative diseases. The value of AI in neurodegenerative diseases becomes more apparent when viewed through the lens of specific case studies, where these techniques are used to enhance detection, improve progression modeling, or optimize treatment approaches. A notable case study is the use of AI in a clinical trial for MCI conducted by [31]. The study proposed using a unique multimodal imaging marker. In an examination of ADNI2 MCI data, the authors used a randomized denoising autoencoder marker (rDAm) as a trial enrichment criterion to minimize the required sample estimates by at least fivefold compared to non-enriched regimes, leading to smaller trials with robust statistical power compared to existing methods, thereby demonstrating the potential of AI for enhancing clinical trials' efficacy.

Another notable example is a systematic review of technical and clinical validation of commercial automated volumetric MRI tools for dementia diagnosis [35]. The evidence on regulatory-approved reports for memory clinics was reviewed, assessing their compliance with the quantitative neuroradiology initiative (QNI) framework. Unbiased technical details of available products were summarized to enhance evidence transparency and present the market's reporting tool variety. Neuroradiologists were employed in making informed decisions on adopting these methods in the clinic. Out of the 17 identified products, 11 companies conducted some technical validation, but only 4 published clinical validation specifically for dementia. The review of published evidence on regulatory-approved reports in dementia highlighted a significant gap in the literature concerning clinical validation, workflow integration, and in-use evaluation for MRI diagnosis in dementia.

Improved performance is commonly achieved by combining multi-modality brain data for disease diagnosis. A multi-modality study utilizing ML techniques to predict cognitive outcomes in individuals with AD Neuroimaging Initiative (ADNI) datasets offered promising results [36]. The authors employed CNNs to predict multi-modality imaging data. The framework's input and output consist of two volumetric modalities. Within the network, numerous trainable parameters captured the relationship between the input and output modalities. By training the network on subjects with all modalities, the authors estimated the output modality based on the input modality. The evaluation was utilizing MRI and PET images as input and output modalities, respectively. The results demonstrated a significant performance improvement compared to previous methods.

In research settings utilizing different raters, it is crucial to establish inter-rater reliability for study assessments. The increasing involvement of advanced practice nurses in tasks traditionally performed by physicians necessitates demonstrating similarity in ratings between nurses and physicians when using assessment tools to ensure confidence among consumers and providers. A case study [37] proposed to establish the inter-rater reliability of neurological assessments conducted by advanced practice nurses and neurologists, which included the Unified PD Rating Scale-Motor Exam. Between August 2007 and January 2008, advanced practice nurses and neurologists independently documented their findings from neurological examinations of 46 participants. The overall agreement between nurse and neurologist ratings was estimated using the intraclass correlation coefficient, while the agreement for individual items on a dichotomous scale was assessed using Cohen's kappa. The results showed substantial agreement between advanced practice nurses and neurologists in their ratings of the Unified PD Rating Scale-Motor Exam and the U.S. National

Alzheimer's Coordinating Center Uniform Data Set neurological examination. These findings supported the conduct of neurological assessments by advanced practice nurses and align with previous studies on the inter-rater agreement of the Unified PD Rating Scale-Motor Exam.

5 Challenges and Limitations in Detecting Neurodegenerative Diseases

5.1 Data Privacy and Security

While AI presents novel opportunities for detecting neurodegenerative diseases, there exist several challenges that need to be addressed before its optimal implementation. These challenges span issues of data privacy and security, interpretability of AI models, potential biases, technological constraints, and ethical and regulatory considerations. In the realm of neurodegenerative disease detection, the deployment of AI brings along the challenge of ensuring data privacy and security, given that the data typically involves sensitive information such as brain scans, genetic profiles, and cognitive scores over time. A prevalent approach to secure privacy, Differential Privacy, implies introducing noise into the query responses, thereby protecting an individual's information [38]. However, the implementation of this approach to neurodegenerative disease detection poses a challenge because it could compromise the accuracy of AI models. Consider a dataset D that consists of patients' medical records and a privacy parameter ε. An algorithm A, which offers ε-differential privacy, would ensure the following condition represented as,

$$P(A(D) = O) \leq e^{\varepsilon} * P(A(D\prime) = O) \tag{7}$$

Here, D' is an adjacent dataset differing by one record. Here, selecting an appropriate ε to maintain data utility while ensuring privacy becomes challenging in the case of neurodegenerative disease detection, as even minor details could be significant. Another concept pertinent to data privacy is k-Anonymity [39], which ensures that an individual's data cannot be distinguished from at least k-1 other individuals in the dataset, represented mathematically as,

$$|\{i \in D \mid D[i, A] = *t*\}| \geq k \tag{8}$$

Here, A is a set of quasi-identifiers, $D[i, A]$ denotes the projection of the tuple i on attributes in A, and t is a combination of quasi-identifier values. The selection of appropriate quasi-identifiers and a suitable k is crucial in the context of neurodegenerative disease detection and a challenge given the wide array of sensitive data.

As the evolution of AI expands the scale and scope of data collected for neurodegenerative disease detection, new privacy concerns emerge. For instance, the use of remote patient monitoring devices and IoT technologies that collect continuous data from patients may exacerbate these privacy issues. Secure Multi-party Computation (SMC) [40] could potentially address these concerns by allowing parties to compute a function over their inputs while keeping those inputs private. However, SMC implementations are computationally intensive and may be difficult to apply in real-world healthcare scenarios.

Given these complexities, it's paramount that robust privacy-preserving mechanisms are devised, and legislation, like the General Data Protection Regulation (GDPR) in the European Union, is strictly adhered to [41]. These privacy laws should guide data collection, processing, and storage activities while ensuring patient consent and privacy. However, harmonizing these regulations globally is another challenge that needs addressing to foster international collaboration in AI-assisted neurodegenerative disease detection. Furthermore, with the rise of quantum computing [42], the threat to encryption algorithms, which currently protect sensitive data, intensifies. Post-quantum cryptography methods need to be explored and implemented to ensure the long-term security of sensitive healthcare data, thereby protecting the privacy rights of patients. While data privacy and security are significant hurdles, they are not insurmountable. A concerted effort from stakeholders, including AI researchers, healthcare professionals, and policymakers, is essential to resolve these challenges and ensure the ethical and secure use of AI in neurodegenerative disease detection. As such, it is evident that advancements in AI should be paralleled with advancements in data privacy and security measures, as this would uphold patient trust and enable the optimal exploitation of AI capabilities in the detection of neurodegenerative diseases.

5.2 *Interpretability of AI Models*

The Interpretability in AI models is a pivotal aspect of clinical acceptance, especially when the predictions of these models are employed for essential decision-making processes. DL models have demonstrated effectiveness in extracting features from neuroimaging data to predict disease progression. However, these models often resemble a *black box*, thereby hindering transparency [43]. The complexity of the interpretability challenge escalates when we consider more sophisticated models such as LSTM networks used for predicting disease progression based on time-series data. Given the multiple elements involved and the temporal dependencies, deciphering how the LSTM uses historical patient data to make future predictions is non-trivial. Techniques like Layer-wise Relevance Propagation (LRP) and Local Interpretable Model-Agnostic Explanations (LIME) [23, 44] can help elucidate the working of these models by attributing the prediction to input features. However, these methods are computationally expensive and may not always yield insights that are easily interpretable to clinicians. Moreover, the nature of neurodegenerative diseases adds another layer of complexity to the interpretability challenge. Neurodegenerative diseases, such as Alzheimer's, involve complex biological processes and are influenced by numerous factors such as genetics, lifestyle, and environmental factors. Therefore, the mapping from input data to disease prediction is inherently complex and may not be fully captured by simple explanatory models.

5.3 Risk of Bias in AI Models

One of the significant challenges with AI models is the risk of propagating or amplifying existing biases in the training data. If not addressed, these biases can result in unequal or incorrect diagnoses, leading to consequential healthcare disparities [45]. Addressing these biases involves various strategies, from collecting diverse and representative data to applying bias mitigation algorithms during model training. It's also important to test the model performance across different subgroups to ensure it generalizes well. To quantify bias in AI models, we often use measures such as the disparate impact ratio (DIR) [46]. DIR measures the likelihood of a positive outcome ($\hat{y} = 1$, such as detecting the disease) for different groups defined by a binary sensitive attribute A (e.g., age, gender, race). The DIR is defined mathematically as,

$$DIR = P(\hat{y} = 1|A = a) / P(\hat{y} = 1|A = \neg a) \tag{9}$$

Here, A is a binary sensitive attribute (e.g., age, gender, race), and a and $\neg a$ represent its possible values. A DIR significantly different from 1 indicates bias, favoring one group over the other. A balanced dataset in terms of these sensitive attributes is crucial to prevent bias in the model's predictions.

Beyond DIR, other metrics also assess different aspects of bias. For instance, Equality of Opportunity (EoO) [45] compares true positive rates between groups, as shown below:

$$EoO = P(\hat{y} = 1 \mid y = 1,\ A = a) / P(\hat{y} = 1 \mid y = 1,\ A = \neg a) \tag{10}$$

Here, y is the ground truth label, and the other symbols retain their meanings from the DIR representation. Like DIR, an EoO value close to 1 signifies a fair model, whereas deviation from 1 implies bias.

Bias in AI models is not limited to sensitive attributes like age, gender, or race. Biases can also occur based on the geographical location where data was collected, which may reflect regional variations in disease prevalence, healthcare practices, or demographics. Similarly, biases can emerge from the type of imaging equipment or imaging protocols used, influencing the model's performance across different clinical settings. Also, selection bias can be introduced if the training data is not representative of the general patient population. For instance, if the training data consists mainly of late-stage disease patients, the model may underperform in detecting early-stage diseases. Such bias can be quantified using metrics such as the Prevalence Index (PI)

[47], defined as,

$$PI = P(y = 1 \mid A = a) \big/ P(y = 1 \mid A = \neg a) \tag{11}$$

Here, y denotes the disease status, and A, a, $\neg a$ have their usual meanings. A PI significantly different from 1 indicates selection bias favoring one group over the other.

5.4 Technological and Resource Limitations

The technological and resource limitations in applying AI to real-world settings arise from computational requirements, data needs, and the integration of AI models with existing healthcare systems. AI, particularly DL models, necessitates substantial computational resources. Training these models involves numerous layers of artificial neurons, each of which needs to process and learn from vast quantities of data. The computational power required scales exponentially with the complexity of the model, rendering it unfeasible for many healthcare settings, especially those in low-resource environments. Let us represent the computational resource required (R) as a function of the number of layers (L), the number of neurons in each layer (N), and the size of the training dataset (D) as shown below:

$$R = C(L, N, D) \tag{12}$$

Here, C is a function representing the computational requirement. For large-scale DL models, C becomes a high-order function, highlighting the surge in computational resource requirements as model complexity increases. The cost of obtaining and maintaining these resources, along with the energy consumption associated, pose significant limitations.

Beyond the computational hurdle, another critical resource limitation is the need for large, high-quality datasets. Data is the lifeblood of AI models, and the quality and quantity of data directly influence the performance and utility of the model. Unfortunately, acquiring large datasets for neurodegenerative diseases is difficult due to patient privacy concerns, the rarity of certain diseases, and data harmonization issues across different healthcare systems. Moreover, the datasets should ideally be diverse, covering different disease stages, demographics, and co-morbidities to ensure a robust and generalizable model.

Another significant technological challenge lies in integrating these AI models with current healthcare systems. Healthcare data is often fragmented across different systems and stored in disparate formats, creating difficulties in data aggregation and interoperability. Even once the models are trained, implementing them for real-time diagnosis in clinical workflows requires seamless integration with existing systems such as EHRs.

The model's deployment also needs to consider the network latency and processing speed, as any delay can have critical consequences in healthcare settings. The processing time (T) can be modeled as a function of the computational resource (R), model complexity (MC), and data input size (S) as shown below:

$$T = P(R, MC, S) \tag{13}$$

Here, P is a function denoting the processing time. It's crucial to optimize this function to minimize latency and ensure real-time processing.

5.5 Ethical and Regulatory Considerations

In the transition towards AI-integrated healthcare, the landscape of neurodegenerative disease detection and management is faced with a myriad of ethical and regulatory considerations. As AI technologies become further embedded in the healthcare sector, the fundamental questions surrounding data privacy, model explainability, inherent bias, and the impact on healthcare professionals intensify. Addressing these queries requires a careful balance of technological innovation, ethical responsibility, and regulatory adaptation [48].

Foremost among these ethical quandaries is data privacy and security. The nature of AI systems necessitates access to large amounts of personal and sensitive health data. However, with this unprecedented access comes the risk of data breaches, misuse, and unauthorized access. Given that neuroimaging data, genetic information, and other medical data used in the detection of neurodegenerative diseases are highly sensitive, the potential harm of a data breach is substantial.

The existing regulatory safeguards, such as the Health Insurance Portability and Accountability Act (HIPAA) in the US, need to evolve to meet these new challenges [49]. Let's denote by $P(D)$ the potential for privacy breach as a function of the size of the dataset (D), security measures in place (S), and the complexity of the AI system (C) used. This can be shown as follows:

$$P(D) = F(D, S, C) \tag{14}$$

Here, F is a function that encapsulates the interplay between the aforementioned parameters. As the size of the dataset increases or if the security measures are inadequate, the potential for a privacy breach escalates, emphasizing the need for rigorous data security measures.

The *black-box* nature of many AI models presents a formidable barrier to their acceptance by healthcare professionals and patients alike. This lack of explainability and transparency impedes the ability to scrutinize and understand the model's decisions, which is essential for clinical acceptance and trust. The development of methods to improve AI interpretability, such as SHAP (Shapley Additive explanations), is critical in addressing this concern [50].

Regulatory considerations also come to the fore as AI technologies make inroads into healthcare. Existing regulations need to be updated and new ones need to be created to keep pace with the rapidly advancing AI field. Regulatory bodies like the FDA are developing guidelines for the validation and use of AI in healthcare [51]. This ongoing regulatory evolution is vital to ensure that AI tools meet rigorous standards of safety and efficacy before their deployment in real-world healthcare settings.

6 Future Perspectives and Opportunities

6.1 AI-Enabled Drug Discovery

AI has emerged as a transformative force in drug discovery, offering a suite of tools that can help circumvent the traditional challenges of drug development in neurodegenerative diseases. Particularly, the application of ML/DL can streamline the drug discovery process, curtail development timelines and costs, and de-risk the process of drug development, catalyzing the progression from bench to bedside [52].

The integral role of AI in drug discovery encapsulates two fundamental aspects—drug target identification and candidate compound discovery [53]. These two processes are traditionally resource-intensive, with a high risk of failure, but the integration of AI can refine and optimize these processes. ML algorithms, such as SVM [54] and random forest (RF), provide the means to sift through massive amounts of genomic, proteomic, and metabolic data, effectively identifying potential disease markers and drug targets associated with neurodegenerative diseases. An SVM, for instance, is particularly adept at binary classification problems, such as distinguishing between disease-related genes and non-disease genes. Furthermore, AI's potential to predict drug-drug interactions and side effects may pave the way for more efficient drug repurposing strategies in neurodegenerative diseases [52].

Following the identification of potential drug targets, AI tools can facilitate the discovery of candidate compounds. ML and DL can parse high-throughput screening data, identify potential therapeutic agents, and predict their properties, such as their absorption, distribution, metabolism, excretion, and toxicity (ADMET) profiles [55]. Let's denote the ADMET properties (P) of a drug as a function of its chemical structure (S) and biological targets (T), as shown below:

$$P = H(S, T) \tag{15}$$

Here, H is a function that encapsulates the relationship between the chemical structure, biological targets, and ADMET properties. The ability of AI to predict these properties allows for the selection of candidate compounds with favorable properties, potentially leading to higher success rates in preclinical and clinical trials.

In the realm of DL, autoencoders and generative models such as Generative Adversarial Networks (GANs) are particularly promising for novel drug discovery [56]. By learning the distribution of drug-like molecules in a high-dimensional latent space, these models can generate novel molecules with desired properties, potentially leading to breakthroughs in the treatment of neurodegenerative diseases. As we continue to refine these AI tools and techniques, the future of drug discovery in neurodegenerative diseases appears increasingly promising.

6.2 Advancements in Neuroimaging and AI

AI holds promise in augmenting the early detection, prognosis, and understanding of neurodegenerative diseases. CNNs have seen successful applications in various neuroimaging modalities, such as magnetic resonance imaging (MRI) and positron emission tomography (PET) scans, enhancing diagnostic accuracy and efficiency. These models are particularly apt for neuroimaging as they can process high-dimensional data, such as images, directly without the need for manual feature extraction. The capacity of AI to handle and analyze vast and complex neuroimaging datasets can elevate diagnostic precision and enable individualized treatment plans for patients with neurodegenerative diseases. Neuroimaging data comprises not only anatomical but also functional, biochemical, and molecular information about the brain. By training AI algorithms on such comprehensive datasets, it's possible to build models that can detect subtle changes in brain structure and function that might be indicative of early-stage neurodegenerative disease [57]. Consider a hypothetical AI system that can output a disease severity score (D) based on an input MRI scan (M). The function could be denoted as follows:

$$D = f(M) \tag{16}$$

Here, f is a highly complex function that the AI system learns to approximate based on a training set of MRI scans and corresponding disease severity scores. This equation highlights how AI can transform raw neuroimaging data into actionable clinical insights.

One of the exciting aspects of AI applications in neuroimaging is their potential to uncover novel insights into the progression and mechanisms of neurodegenerative diseases. Advanced AI models can process neuroimaging data over time to create a dynamic picture of disease progression and potentially identify new patterns or markers of these diseases [58]. Furthermore, AI algorithms could unveil relationships between various biomarkers, both within and across different modalities, yielding a more comprehensive understanding of disease pathophysiology. Moreover, the integration of AI and neuroimaging could fuel advancements in the design of clinical trials for new treatments. AI models could assist in participant selection by identifying patients who are most likely to benefit from a particular treatment based on their neuroimaging data. This could not only increase the efficiency of trials but also enhance their ethical profile by minimizing exposure to potential risks among those less likely to benefit.

Integrating AI with neuroimaging also opens up the possibility of predictive modeling, whereby AI could forecast disease progression based on current and past neuroimaging data. Such predictive models could assist in patient counseling, care planning, and therapeutic decision-making [59]. Further, transfer learning is a promising method in the AI-neuroimaging domain. Transfer learning techniques allow the application of knowledge learned from one problem domain to another, facilitating the development of robust models even when the target domain has limited data [12]. For instance, an AI model trained to identify features in MRI scans related to Alzheimer's disease might apply that knowledge to the detection of related neurodegenerative conditions like vascular dementia.

The synergistic integration of AI and neuroimaging presents an exciting horizon in neurodegenerative disease research, promising more accurate diagnoses, personalized treatments, novel insights into disease mechanisms, efficient clinical trials, and improved care planning. Despite these significant strides, the complexity and sensitivity of neuroimaging data mandate rigorous testing and validation of AI algorithms to ensure reliable and ethical use. As research progresses, the future of neurodegenerative disease detection and treatment looks increasingly bright, thanks to the powerful alliance of AI and neuroimaging.

7 Conclusion

In concluding this comprehensive overview of AI in neurodegenerative diseases, it is evident that AI presents a transformative opportunity for the diagnosis, management, and treatment of such conditions. A broad and nuanced landscape of AI's role in healthcare and specifically in neurodegenerative diseases has been traversed in this chapter, providing insights into the historical, current, and potential future implications of AI in this critical medical arena.

From the early instances of AI applications in medical diagnosis to the complex DL models in use today, we have seen a remarkable progression in AI's capabilities. The different AI techniques, such as supervised, unsupervised, reinforcement, and other advanced algorithms, have been mathematically and theoretically analyzed, thereby illuminating their multifaceted utility in discerning and combatting neurodegenerative diseases. The current state of AI applications in neurodegenerative diseases underscores a promising trajectory, from facilitating early disease detection and diagnosis to modeling disease progression and informing personalized treatment plans. AI's potential extends even further into drug discovery and advancements in neuroimaging, potentially revolutionizing these aspects of healthcare.

However, the promise of AI is not without its challenges. As discussed, the hurdles in data privacy and security, interpretability of AI models, risk of bias, and technological and resource limitations, pose significant obstacles. Notably, these challenges have mathematical and technical implications that affect the design, implementation, and deployment of AI models in the healthcare sector. With advancements come critical ethical and regulatory considerations. AI's transformative potential must be coupled with robust ethical frameworks and regulatory guidelines to ensure the safe, equitable, and effective deployment of these technologies. These considerations span data privacy, algorithmic transparency, and potential biases, underscoring the need for interdisciplinary collaboration to address these multidimensional challenges.

In light of these insights, it is clear that the future of AI in neurodegenerative diseases is one of both promise and complexity. The road to fully integrating AI into neurodegenerative disease care is long and winding, filled with both enormous potential and significant challenges. Yet, with the insights presented in this chapter and the collaborative efforts of researchers, healthcare professionals, technologists, ethicists, and regulators, AI's promise in neurodegenerative diseases can be fulfilled, thereby ushering in a new era of healthcare that leverages the best of technology to improve patient outcomes and advance our understanding of these complex diseases.

Despite the progress in understanding the intricate mechanisms underpinning neurodegenerative diseases, numerous challenges lie ahead. Future research needs to delve deeper into the exact causes of these diseases, identify reliable biomarkers for early detection and prognosis, and develop effective strategies to halt or reverse neurodegeneration. A multidisciplinary approach, incorporating genetics, molecular biology, neuroscience, and pharmacology, is essential to achieve this goal.

As we continue to refine these technologies and delve deeper into the potential of AI, we must remember that our primary goal is to improve patient care and outcomes. Whether through enhancing diagnosis accuracy, discovering new potential therapeutic agents, or refining our understanding of disease progression, our efforts must always align with this mission. The interplay of AI in neurodegenerative diseases is a burgeoning field that presents a compelling intersection of technology, medicine, and ethics. This chapter has sought to provide a comprehensive exploration of this critical field, capturing its opportunities, challenges, and future perspectives. It is a testament to the evolving narrative of AI in healthcare—a narrative that we must continue to shape with due diligence, ethical considerations, and above all, a commitment to improving patient care in neurodegenerative diseases.

References

1. Lynch, S., Andrew Ng: Why AI is the new electricity, https://news.stanford.edu/thedish/2017/03/14/andrew-ng-why-ai-is-the-new-electricity/.
2. Erkkinen, M. G., Kim, M.-O., & Geschwind, M. D. (2018). Clinical neurology and epidemiology of the major neurodegenerative diseases. *Cold Spring Harbor Perspectives Biology, 10.* https://doi.org/10.1101/cshperspect.a033118.
3. Jellinger, K. A. (2010). Basic mechanisms of neurodegeneration: A critical update. *Journal of Cellular and Molecular Medicine, 14*, 457–487. https://doi.org/10.1111/j.1582-4934.2010.01010.x
4. Ross, C. A., & Poirier, M. A. (2004). Protein aggregation and neurodegenerative disease. *Nature Medicine, 10*(Suppl), S10–S17. https://doi.org/10.1038/nm1066

5. Glass, C. K., Saijo, K., Winner, B., Marchetto, M. C., & Gage, F. H. (2010). Mechanisms underlying inflammation in neurodegeneration. *Cell, 140*, 918–934. https://doi.org/10.1016/j.cell.2010.02.016
6. Dias, V., Junn, E., & Mouradian, M. M. (2013). The role of oxidative stress in Parkinson's disease. *Journal of Parkinson's Disease, 3*, 461–491. https://doi.org/10.3233/JPD-130230
7. Shortliffe, E. H., & Buchanan, B. G. (1975). A model of inexact reasoning in medicine. *Mathematical Bioscience, 23*, 351–379. https://doi.org/10.1016/0025-5564(75)90047-4.
8. Lindsay, R. K., Buchanan, B. G., Feigenbaum, E. A., & Lederberg, J. (1993). DENDRAL: A case study of the first expert system for scientific hypothesis formation. *Artificial Intelligent, 61*, 209–261. https://doi.org/10.1016/0004-3702(93)90068-M.
9. Miller, R. A., Pople, H. E. J., & Myers, J. D. (1982). Internist-1, an experimental computer-based diagnostic consultant for general internal medicine. *New England Journal of Medicine, 307*, 468–476. https://doi.org/10.1056/NEJM198208193070803
10. de Dombal, F. T., Leaper, D. J., Staniland, J. R., McCann, A. P., & Horrocks, J. C. (1972). Computer-aided diagnosis of acute abdominal pain. *British Medical Journal, 2*, 9 LP—13. https://doi.org/10.1136/bmj.2.5804.9.
11. Sharma, N., Sharma, R., & Jindal, N. (2021). Machine learning and deep learning applications-a vision. *Global Transitions Proceedings, 2*, 24–28. https://doi.org/10.1016/j.gltp.2021.01.004.
12. Litjens, G., Kooi, T., Bejnordi, B. E., Setio, A. A. A., Ciompi, F., Ghafoorian, M., van der Laak, J. A. W. M., van Ginneken, B., & Sánchez, C. I. (2017). A survey on deep learning in medical image analysis. *Medical Image Analysis, 42*, 60–88. https://doi.org/10.1016/j.media.2017.07.005.
13. Esteva, A., Kuprel, B., Novoa, R. A., Ko, J., Swetter, S. M., Blau, H. M., & Thrun, S. (2017). Dermatologist-level classification of skin cancer with deep neural networks. *Nature, 542*, 115–118. https://doi.org/10.1038/nature21056
14. De Fauw, J., Ledsam, J. R., Romera-Paredes, B., Nikolov, S., Tomasev, N., Blackwell, S., Askham, H., Glorot, X., O'Donoghue, B., Visentin, D., van den Driessche, G., Lakshminarayanan, B., Meyer, C., Mackinder, F., Bouton, S., Ayoub, K., Chopra, R., King, D., Karthikesalingam, A., … Ronneberger, O. (2018). Clinically applicable deep learning for diagnosis and referral in retinal disease. *Nature Medicine, 24*, 1342–1350. https://doi.org/10.1038/s41591-018-0107-6
15. Obermeyer, Z., & Emanuel, E. J. (2016). Predicting the future—big data, machine learning, and clinical medicine. *New England Journal of Medicine, 375*, 1216–1219. https://doi.org/10.1056/NEJMp1606181
16. Raghupathi, W., & Raghupathi, V. (2014). Big data analytics in healthcare: Promise and potential. *Health Information Science System, 2*, 3. https://doi.org/10.1186/2047-2501-2-3
17. Verdejo Espinosa, Á., Lopez Ruiz, J., Mata Mata, F., & Estevez, M. E. (2021). Application of IoT in healthcare: Keys to implementation of the sustainable development goals. *Sensors, 21*. https://doi.org/10.3390/s21072330.
18. Alzubaidi, L., Zhang, J., Humaidi, A. J., Al-Dujaili, A., Duan, Y., Al-Shamma, O., Santamaría, J., Fadhel, M. A., Al-Amidie, M., & Farhan, L. (2021). *Review of deep learning: concepts, CNN architectures, challenges, applications, future directions*. Springer International Publishing (2021).https://doi.org/10.1186/s40537-021-00444-8
19. Pyrros, A., Rodriguez Fernandez, J., Borstelmann, S. M., Flanders, A., Wenzke, D., Hart, E., Horowitz, J. M., Nikolaidis, P., Willis, M., Chen, A., Cole, P., Siddiqui, N., Muzaffar, M., Muzaffar, N., McVean, J., Menchaca, M., Katsaggelos, A. K., Koyejo, S., & Galanter, W. (2022). Validation of a deep learning, value-based care model to predict mortality and comorbidities from chest radiographs in COVID-19. *PLOS Digital Health, 1*, e0000057. https://doi.org/10.1371/journal.pdig.0000057
20. Wang, L., Li, P., Hou, M., Zhang, X., Cao, X., & Li, H. (2021). Construction of a risk prediction model for Alzheimer's disease in the elderly population. *BMC Neurology, 21*, 271. https://doi.org/10.1186/s12883-021-02276-8
21. Rasmussen, C. E., & Williams, C. K. I. (2004). *Gaussian processes for machine learning*.https://doi.org/10.1142/S0129065704001899

22. Vichianin, Y., Khummongkol, A., Chiewvit, P., Raksthaput, A., Chaichanettee, S., Aoonkaew, N., & Senanarong, V. (2021). Accuracy of support-vector machines for diagnosis of Alzheimer's disease, using volume of brain obtained by structural MRI at Siriraj Hospital. *Frontiers Neurology, 12*. https://doi.org/10.3389/fneur.2021.640696.
23. Samek, W., Binder, A., Montavon, G., Lapuschkin, S., & Müller, K. R. (2017). Evaluating the visualization of what a deep neural network has learned. *IEEE Transactions on Neural Networks Learning System, 28*, 2660–2673. https://doi.org/10.1109/TNNLS.2016.2599820
24. Habes, M., Grothe, M. J., Tunc, B., McMillan, C., Wolk, D. A., & Davatzikos, C. (2020). Disentangling heterogeneity in Alzheimer's disease and related dementias using data-driven methods. *Biological Psychiatry, 88*, 70–82. https://doi.org/10.1016/j.biopsych.2020.01.016
25. Mnih, V., Kavukcuoglu, K., Silver, D., Rusu, A. A., Veness, J., Bellemare, M. G., Graves, A., Riedmiller, M., Fidjeland, A. K., Ostrovski, G., Petersen, S., Beattie, C., Sadik, A., Antonoglou, I., King, H., Kumaran, D., Wierstra, D., Legg, S., & Hassabis, D. (2015). Human-level control through deep reinforcement learning. *Nature, 518*, 529–533. https://doi.org/10.1038/nature14236
26. Khaliq, F., Oberhauser, J., Wakhloo, D., & Mahajani, S. (2023). Decoding degeneration: The implementation of machine learning for clinical detection of neurodegenerative disorders. *Neural Regeneration Research, 18*, 1235–1242. https://doi.org/10.4103/1673-5374.355982
27. Myszczynska, M. A., Ojamies, P. N., Lacoste, A. M. B., Neil, D., Saffari, A., Mead, R., Hautbergue, G. M., Holbrook, J. D., & Ferraiuolo, L. (2020). Applications of machine learning to diagnosis and treatment of neurodegenerative diseases. *Nature Reviews Neurology, 16*, 440–456. https://doi.org/10.1038/s41582-020-0377-8
28. Liu, M., Cheng, D., & Yan, W. (2018). Initiative, Alzheimer's Disease neuroimaging: Classification of Alzheimer's disease by combination of convolutional and recurrent neural networks using FDG-PET images. *Frontiers Neuroinformation, 12*. https://doi.org/10.3389/fninf.2018.00035.
29. Hochreiter, S., & Schmidhuber, J. (1997). Long short-term memory. *Neural Computation, 9*, 1735–1780. https://doi.org/10.1162/neco.1997.9.8.1735
30. Zhang, D., Shen, D., & Initiative, A. D. N. (2012). Predicting future clinical changes of MCI patients using longitudinal and multimodal biomarkers. *PLoS ONE, 7*, 1–15. https://doi.org/10.1371/journal.pone.0033182
31. Ithapu, V. K., Singh, V., Okonkwo, O. C., Chappell, R. J., Dowling, N. M., & Johnson, S. C. (2015). Imaging-based enrichment criteria using deep learning algorithms for efficient clinical trials in mild cognitive impairment. *Alzheimer's & Dementia, 11*, 1489–1499. https://doi.org/10.1016/j.jalz.2015.01.010
32. Sarraf, S., & Tofighi, G. (2016). *Classification of Alzheimer's disease using fMRI data and deep learning convolutional neural networks.*
33. Ali, L., Zhu, C., Zhang, Z., & Liu, Y. (2019). Automated detection of Parkinson's disease based on multiple types of sustained phonations using linear discriminant analysis and genetically optimized neural network. *IEEE Journal Translational Engineering Health Medical, 7*, 2000410. https://doi.org/10.1109/JTEHM.2019.2940900
34. Keine, D., Walker, J. Q., Kennedy, B. K., & Sabbagh, M. N. (2018). Development, application, and results from a precision-medicine platform that personalizes multi-modal treatment plans for Mild Alzheimer's disease and At-risk individuals. *Current Aging Science, 11*, 173–181. https://doi.org/10.2174/1874609811666181019101430
35. Pemberton, H. G., Zaki, L. A. M., Goodkin, O., Das, R. K., Steketee, R. M. E., Barkhof, F., & Vernooij, M. W. (2021). Technical and clinical validation of commercial automated volumetric MRI tools for dementia diagnosis—a systematic review. *Neuroradiology, 63*, 1773–1789. https://doi.org/10.1007/s00234-021-02746-3
36. Li, R., Zhang, W., Suk, H.-I., Wang, L., Li, J., Shen, D., & Ji, S. (2014). Deep learning based imaging data completion for improved brain disease diagnosis. Med. image Comput. Comput. Interv. MICCAI ... *International Conference Medical Image Computing and Computer Interaction, 17*, 305–312. https://doi.org/10.1007/978-3-319-10443-0_39.

37. Palmer, J. L., Coats, M. A., Roe, C. M., Hanko, S. M., Xiong, C., & Morris, J. C. (2010). Unified Parkinson's disease rating scale-motor exam: Inter-rater reliability of advanced practice nurse and neurologist assessments. *Journal of Advanced Nursing, 66*, 1382–1387. https://doi.org/10.1111/j.1365-2648.2010.05313.x
38. Dyda, A., Purcell, M., Curtis, S., Field, E., Pillai, P., Ricardo, K., Weng, H., Moore, J. C., Hewett, M., Williams, G., & Lau, C. L. (2021). Differential privacy for public health data: An innovative tool to optimize information sharing while protecting data confidentiality. Patterns (New York, N.Y.). 2, 100366 (2021). https://doi.org/10.1016/j.patter.2021.100366.
39. Sweeney, L. (2022). K-Anonymity: A model for protecting privacy. *International Journal Uncertain. Fuzziness Knowledge-Based System 10*, 557–570. https://doi.org/10.1142/S0218488502001648.
40. Frikken, K. B. (2011). Secure multiparty computation (SMC). In H. C. A. van Tilborg & S. Jajodia (eds.) *Encyclopedia of Cryptography and Security*. pp. 1121–1123. Springer US, Boston, MA. https://doi.org/10.1007/978-1-4419-5906-5_766.
41. Mondschein, C. F., & Monda, C. (2019). The EU's general data protection regulation (GDPR) in a research context. In P. Kubben, M. Dumontier & A. Dekker (eds.) *Fundamentals of Clinical Data Science*, pp. 55–71. Springer International Publishing, Cham. https://doi.org/10.1007/978-3-319-99713-1_5.
42. Rietsche, R., Dremel, C., Bosch, S., Steinacker, L., Meckel, M., & Leimeister, J.-M. (2022). Quantum computing. *Electronic Markets, 32*, 2525–2536. https://doi.org/10.1007/s12525-022-00570-y
43. Kermany, D. S., Goldbaum, M., Cai, W., Valentim, C. C. S., Liang, H., Baxter, S. L., McKeown, A., Yang, G., Wu, X., Yan, F., Dong, J., Prasadha, M. K., Pei, J., Ting, M., Zhu, J., Li, C., Hewett, S., Dong, J., Ziyar, I., … Zhang, K. (2018). Identifying medical diagnoses and treatable diseases by image-based deep learning. *Cell, 172*, 1122-1124.e9. https://doi.org/10.1016/j.cell.2018.02.010
44. Kim, I., Rajaraman, S., & Antani, S. (2019). Visual interpretation of convolutional neural network predictions in classifying medical image modalities. Diagnostics. https://doi.org/10.3390/diagnostics9020038
45. Rajkomar, A., Hardt, M., Howell, M. D., Corrado, G., & Chin, M. H. (2018). Ensuring fairness in machine learning to advance health equity. *Annals of Internal Medicine, 169*, 866–872. https://doi.org/10.7326/M18-1990
46. Feldman, M., Friedler, S. A., Moeller, J., Scheidegger, C., & Venkatasubramanian, S. (2015). Certifying and removing disparate impact. In *Proceedings of the 21th ACM SIGKDD International Conference on Knowledge Discovery and Data Mining*, pp. 259–268. Association for Computing Machinery, New York, NY, USA. https://doi.org/10.1145/2783258.2783311.
47. Christie, A. P., Abecasis, D., Adjeroud, M., Alonso, J. C., Amano, T., Anton, A., Baldigo, B. P., Barrientos, R., Bicknell, J. E., Buhl, D. A., Cebrian, J., Ceia, R. S., Cibils-Martina, L., Clarke, S., Claudet, J., Craig, M. D., Davoult, D., De Backer, A., Donovan, M. K., … Sutherland, W. J. (2020). Quantifying and addressing the prevalence and bias of study designs in the environmental and social sciences. *Nature Communications, 11*, 6377. https://doi.org/10.1038/s41467-020-20142-y
48. Mittelstadt, B. D., Allo, P., Taddeo, M., Wachter, S., & Floridi, L. (2016). The ethics of algorithms: Mapping the debate. *Big Data and Social 3*, 2053951716679679. https://doi.org/10.1177/2053951716679679.
49. McGraw, D. (2013). Building public trust in uses of health insurance portability and accountability act de-identified data. *Journal of the American Medical Informatics Association, 20*, 29–34. https://doi.org/10.1136/amiajnl-2012-000936
50. Rodríguez-Pérez, R., & Bajorath, J. (2020). Interpretation of machine learning models using shapley values: Application to compound potency and multi-target activity predictions. *Journal of Computer-Aided Molecular Design, 34*, 1013–1026. https://doi.org/10.1007/s10822-020-00314-0
51. Shah, P., Kendall, F., Khozin, S., Goosen, R., Hu, J., Laramie, J., Ringel, M., & Schork, N. (2019). Artificial intelligence and machine learning in clinical development: A translational perspective. *npj Digital Media, 2*, 69. https://doi.org/10.1038/s41746-019-0148-3.

52. Vamathevan, J., Clark, D., Czodrowski, P., Dunham, I., Ferran, E., Lee, G., Li, B., Madabhushi, A., Shah, P., Spitzer, M., & Zhao, S. (2019). Applications of machine learning in drug discovery and development. *Nature Reviews. Drug Discovery, 18*, 463–477. https://doi.org/10.1038/s41573-019-0024-5
53. Dara, S., Dhamercherla, S., Jadav, S. S., Babu, C. H. M., & Ahsan, M. J. (2022). Machine learning in drug discovery: A review. *Artificial Intelligence Review, 55*, 1947–1999. https://doi.org/10.1007/s10462-021-10058-4
54. Noble, W. S. (2006). What is a support vector machine? *Nature Biotechnology, 24*, 1565–1567. https://doi.org/10.1038/nbt1206-1565
55. Jia, L., & Gao, H. (2022). Machine learning for In Silico ADMET prediction. *Methods in Molecular Biology, 2390*, 447–460. https://doi.org/10.1007/978-1-0716-1787-8_20
56. Abbasi, M., Santos, B. P., Pereira, T. C., Sofia, R., Monteiro, N. R. C., Simões, C. J. V, Brito, R. M. M., Ribeiro, B., Oliveira, J. L., & Arrais, J. P. (2022). Designing optimized drug candidates with Generative Adversarial Network. *Journal Cheminformation, 14*, 40. https://doi.org/10.1186/s13321-022-00623-6.
57. Bhatele, K. R., Jha, A., Kapoor, K., & Tiwari, D. (2022). Neurodegenerative diseases-Caps: A capsule network based early screening system for the classification of neurodegenerative diseases. *Cognitive Neurodynamics, 16*, 1361–1377. https://doi.org/10.1007/s11571-022-09787-1
58. Counts, S. E., Ikonomovic, M. D., Mercado, N., Vega, I. E., & Mufson, E. J. (2017). Biomarkers for the early detection and progression of Alzheimer's disease. *Neurotherapeutics, 14*, 35–53. https://doi.org/10.1007/s13311-016-0481-z
59. Kormas, P., & Moutzouri, A. (2020). Current psychological approaches in neurodegenerative diseases. In P. Vlamos, I. S. Kotsireas, & I. Tarnanas (eds.) *Handbook of Computational Neurodegeneration*, pp. 1–29. Springer International Publishing, Cham. https://doi.org/10.1007/978-3-319-75479-6_10-1.

AI Enhancing Digital Communication in Neurodegenerative Disease Treatment

Kavita Thapliyal and Manjul Thapliyal

Abstract Artificial Intelligence is rapidly transforming the healthcare industry by facilitating healthcare users with innovative digital products which are data driven, easy to use and accurate. These advanced AI enabled systems bring multiple benefits along like reducing cost and administrative load as well as enhancing service, monitoring and treatment facilitation. Cognitive health is one of the major areas of medical and social concern and Artificial Intelligence is playing a vital role in revolutionizing the medical and diagnostic field (Julie and Chow, Prediction of neurodevelopmental disorders based on de novo coding variation. Springer, [14]). Intellectual Disability (ID), Development Disability (DD) and autism spectrum disorder (ASD) are some of the Neuro Degenerative Disorders involving multiple health complications where nervous system and cells are damaged beyond control to seriously impact strength, sensation, mobility, speech, memory, cognition, and coordination in a human body. NDD affects millions of people globally and there is no comprehensive cure for most of these complex diseases. The cost of Neuro Degenerative treatment is extremely costly globally so the need for cost-effective innovative technology is vital to deal diligently with this critical health issue. Modern research and technology are improving by the day to offer new treatments, prognosis, remedies, recurrence risk evaluation and rehabilitation programs that enhance medical systems in the related NDD field to improve patients' mobility, speech and sensation through therapies, exercises and medication to make a notable difference in the quality life of the patient and their family member (Alyssa Blesson, Cold Spring Horbor, [1]). This chapter will try to cover the role of AI in enabling NDD facilitation, apart from introspecting. Also, AI's positive roles, critical areas, hindrances, risks, and scope of improvement with advancement of technology coordinated with Neuro Diseases will be explained in detail.

K. Thapliyal (✉)
Amity International Business School, Amity University, Noida, India
e-mail: kthapliyal@amity.edu

M. Thapliyal
Social Impact Consultant, Visions Ahead Foundation, Noida, India

© The Author(s), under exclusive license to Springer Nature Switzerland AG 2024

L. Gaur et al. (eds.), *AI and Neuro-Degenerative Diseases*, Studies in Computational Intelligence 1131, https://doi.org/10.1007/978-3-031-53148-4_9

Keywords Neurodegenerative diseases · Artificial intelligence · Machine learning · Deep learning · Neural networks · NDDs · Biomarkers · Progressive diseases · Diagnosis · Cognitive · Co- Morbidities · Neurological disorders · Alzheimer's · Parkinsons · Dementia · Cybersecurity · Healthcare · Privacy

1 Introduction

1.1 Neuro Degenerative Disorder

NDD or Neuro Degenerative Disorder is related to the brain where some of the cells of the brain become damaged or dead over a period. Neuro Degeneration can lead to irrevocable neuronal loss leading to death at times. This continuous loss and degradation of neurons and glial cells lead to degradation of spine and brain. This can lead to serious health issues like lack of coordination, balance and speech called Ataxias, which causes difficulty in walking, steadiness and speaking. It can also cause Dementias, leading to loss of cognitive functions affecting thinking, reasoning ad remembering in humans. It hampers a person's mental functioning and weakens his ability to speak, move and breathe further. Neuro Degenerative Diseases are almost incurable and mostly prevalent among the elderly population, leading to adverse effects among families. Some of the common Neuro Degenerative Disorders are Alzheimer's, Parkinson's, Ataxia, Synucleinopathies, Prion, Huntington's, Spinal Muscular Atrophy, Multiple System Atrophy, Progressive Supranuclear Palsy and Motor Neuron Diseases. Such patients require extremely elevated level of patient handling and care as these disorders are progressive and chronic. They lead to motor dysfunction, cognitive decline, thus severely affecting the nervous system and often leading to premature death. As per reliable sources, Dementia globally affects more than fifty million people alone. Artificial Intelligence is positively revolutionizing the understanding, diagnosis, and treatment of neurodegenerative diseases along with new opportunities and challenges associated with it. In the study by [5] states the understanding of the risk factors linked to NDD and they in detailed studied the risk factors database of NDD including 998 single using 2293 records and 1071 articles that all discussed about the concerns of NDD. It was noted that AI and Explainable AI-XAI is going to be the most used and meaningful technology to smartly diagnose and prevent NDDs (Fig. 1).

The chapter will deliberate on the futuristic projections and limitations that Neurogenerative Diseases and Artificial Intelligence will propose when working in tandem. Also there will be analysis on the diversified types of NDs and their clinical indicators [3]. The role of AI must be assessed in detecting and sensing the Neurogenerative Disesases accurately with the help of imaging systems and machine learning algorithms which include advanced techniques Positron Emission Tomography (PET), Magnetic Resonance Imaging (MRI), Recovery Oriented Cognitive Therapy (CT-R)

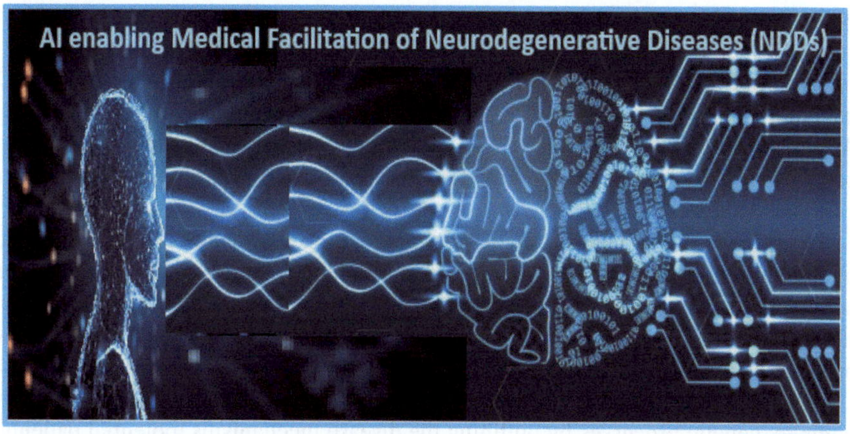

Fig. 1 AI enabling medical facilitation of NDDs

and Cognitive Behavioural Therapy for Psychosis (CBTp). The use of AI in the detection of drugs and the probability to be used for tailored medicine will be explored in detail. The challenges arising due to integration of AI with NDDs has been outlined such as, the imminent requirement of huge, diversified datasets, and the hindrances in understanding the algorithms of AI and its principled consequences in the healthcare sector. Also discussed are the vitality of effective alliances between medical researchers, data scientists and clinic operators to warrant, all round development and real-life impact due to practical implementation of NDDs with AI.

Comprehensively the implementation of AI to counter NDDs is a significant breakthrough in the corrective diagnosis, treatment and overall management of these health draining disorders. Its however vital to carefully consider the clinical, technical, ethical, and mental implications of the persistent use of this digital technology. The chapter aims to explore modern development and research in AI design and deployment of Neuroscience systems and techniques to integrate related theories, applications, methodologies, and real-world experiences and applications leading to breakthrough technologies for NDDs. The comprehensive viewpoint from researchers, scientists, reviewers, industry professions are to be collaborated for real world experiences and indigenous digital products.

2 Positive Prospects of AI Enabling Neuro Degenerative Disorders

Initial Finding and Diagnosis: AI is enabling NDDs greatly with early detections and further in corrective diagnosis by analysing huge pool of datasets of patient's medical history, images, genomic informatics and integral reproducible biomarkers [25] to classify forms that can forecast the early start and monitor of neurodegenerative diseases before symptoms showcase (Fig. 2).

Personal Tailored Medicine: AI helps in deep predictive analysis of NDD patient's medical history based on diversified indicators like CoMorbidities Health Appraisals, Lifestyles, Genetics and Environmental Impacts, thus providing a comprehensive and personalized medical toolkit to cater to irrevocable and multi complex disorders.

Drug Research & Development: With AI playing crucial and critical role in the treatment of NDDs, there is ample acceleration in the research and development of suitable drugs needed to treat the disorders. Suitably predicting targeted candidates, interactions, and drug treatment as per personal analysis and optimized drug designs are steps in progressive treatment of the patient.

Apt Modelling of the Disease: AI can help in NDD treatment by easing out complex genetic processes by outlining the disease mechanisms, potential patients, heredity integrations and its further rejuvenation and treatment progressions.

Close Monitoring of Patients: AI enabled devises and digital support systems integrated through Machine & Deep Learning (ML & DL) help in close monitoring of body and health parameters. The positioning of artificial intelligence (AI) and machine learning (ML) models has been instrumental in neurodegenerative disorder diagnosis. These models help in enhancing diagnostic precision, lowering the strain on healthcare systems, and eventually enhancing the well-being of patients [16]. Instant monitoring tools, wearable devices, patient medical history analysis play a key role in tracking the health progressions of NDD on a timely basis and change the treatment plan as per results of the patients [4]. Wearable AI has immense potential due to its unique features and smart alignments through any electronic device with bracelets, watches, clothes and many apparels and accessories. Precision medicine will cooperate a strategic role toward a specified method required to treat complicated neurodegenerative diseases. From past few years this has been steadily gaining

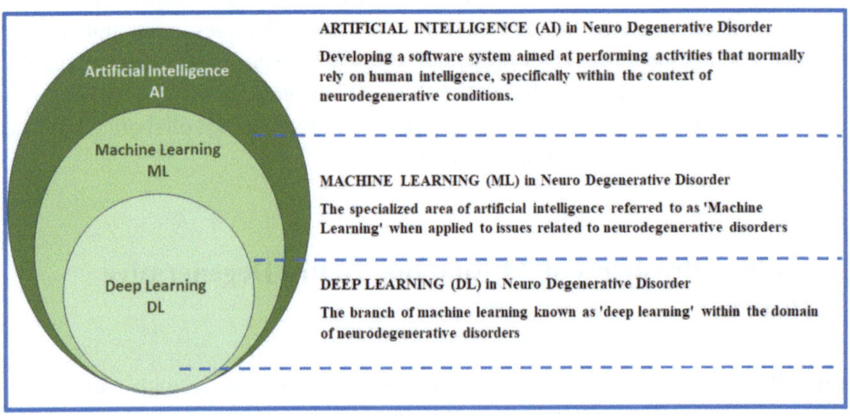

Fig. 2 Positive prospects of AI enabling NDDs

power that artificial intelligence is going to create immense positive influence in treating NDD [7]. In the recent study [17] Alzheimer's disease could only be diagnosed postmortem through brain autopsies. However, since the early 2000s, developments in research have supported the finding of disease signs and the exploration of treatments years before symptoms manifest. By the help of AI modern diagnostic tools like positron emission tomography (PET) brain imaging and cerebrospinal fluid (CSF) tests now support in the before time diagnosis of Alzheimer's disease. Neurodegenerative diseases are a group of disorders described by the radical loss of structure and function of neurons in the brain that are directly associated with cognitive impairment and/or motor dysfunction. The prevalence of neurodegenerative diseases is also increasing due to aging population [15], and currently, there are no effective treatments for most neurodegenerative diseases. AI has the potential to transform the field of neurodegenerative diseases by providing new understandings into disease machineries, enabling earlier and more precise diagnosis, envisaging disease progression, and identifying new targets for drug development.

3 AI Challenges in Neuro Degenerative Disorders

1. **Handling Data Quantity and Quality**: For making precise and timely forecasts, AI algorithms often depend on huge and good quality datasets. But in Neurodegenerative research and development, there may be scarcity of data, or the database may be of inferior quality, thus having major difficulties in further training AI Models.

Ethical Integrations:

2. The NDD treatment tools, systems and diagnostics equipment's will always have to ethically measure queries relating to privacy of data, consent approval, and impartiality in care access.
3. **Compliance & Regulation Hiccups**: The new generation drugs, systems and medical digital devices enabled by AI must surpass numerous testing measures, compliance, and statutory regulations before being put to any clinical practical usage.
4. **Interpretation**: Interpretability of AI systems and models can be intricate and complex to make predictions making it difficult to access their ways of making forecasts. Thus, lacking in transparency, they raise numerous doubts which can be a big hindrance in its research and final adaption in clinical adaptability.
5. **Mapping and Integrating with existing Healthcare systems**: One of the most crucial aspects of AI powered tools in NDD is perfect mapping and integration of the novel tools with existing systems which at times can be critical, intricate and time oriented. AI is making breakthrough technologies in Biomedicine, Bio Medical Engineering and Healthcare Sector.

Apart from the above challenges, there are many other hindrances which need to be taken care of while integrating AI applications with NDDs.

1. **Disease Diversity**: On of the major challenges in NDDs is its heterogeneity which makes the disease complex due to various diversity it carries along. This leads to varied symptoms, multiple health issues, disease development and other fundamental symptoms may differ from patient to patient. The algorithms of AI are not tuned to handle high variance and multiple data sets to predict the diagnosis accurately to further treat the patients.
2. **Complex Data Quality & Quantity**: The major problem is obtaining huge datasets which are of reliable and good quality which are a must while AI handles NDDs as it solely relies on them to predict its results accurately which will further lead towards effective treatment and diagnosis processes. NDDs being rare and complex diseases make it further difficult to obtain correct and precise data. This is otherwise of high cost as research and analyzation of brains condition by biomarkers and brain imaging is a tedious and complex process.
3. **Validity at Clinical Channels**: The safety and validity of any complex testing tool or systems depends on its compliances and clinical validations to ensure patients safety and products effectiveness. AI must integrate seamlessly with neurodegenerative diseases then only the diagnostics and therapeutic tools will be in complete sync. To validate the same, there must be close synchronization between academia, industry, and compliance & regulatory bodies.
4. **Clinical Practice Amalgamations**: Integration of AI tools into clinical practice is of major importance and a critical challenge even if they are at the primitive stage showing positive results. Regular changes in medical practices and government policies are vital as is intricate training of professionals to handle the new age digital technology and complex NDDs functionalities.

Ethical Implications:

5. NDDs are extremely sensitive and critical medical entities, which require very personal and human touch healings. Patient Privacy, data security, proper consent, biases of any form and sensitive information is of utmost importance and needs proper risk mitigation strategies. Ethical touch is foremost here and AI using patients predictive testing vitals are very delicate data's which can severely impact patient's profession, personality, and insurability. Since patient's personal data is involved and used for research there may be legal compliance issues of proper patient consent.

Thus, AI tools integration with NDDs shows incredible scope and vast potential in handling the critical disease diagnostics, therapeutic approaches, and personalised treatment smoothly and ethically [6]. The challenges in integration must be properly mapped and measured taking the technology to its best usage, true potential, and logical conclusion. Medical entities, researchers, industry professionals, scientists must effectively align and introspect on the challenges and further aid in developing of AI as a safe, ethical, and easily accessible potent tool for the masses.

The Neurodegenerative diseases are an aligned group of progressive and critical medical disorders that hamper and degrade the nervous system leading to advanced and regular loss of neurons and their related functionality. The disease is marked by intricate characters like cellular variations and accumulated concentration of abnormal proteins leading to decline in cognitive skills, motor dysfunction and finally death.

4 The More Popular Neuro Degenerative Disorders Are

1. **Parkinsons Disease**: One of the most common and fastest growing NDDs is Parkinson, which is a progressive neurological ailment. The nerve cells start malfunctioning and produce fewer chemical dopamine leaving them confused and not able to recognize things or do things on their own. Substantia Nigra or degeneration of the nerve cells causes loss of control in movements and postures and causes rigidity and tremors.
2. **Alzheimer's**: Cognitive and impairment in behaviour is observed in this neurodegenerative disorder hampering occupational and social functions. This progressive disorder is largely irredeemable. With loss of memory and thinking skills, people are unable to complete even the simplest of tasks. It mostly affects people of sixty-five plus age group and is also the most common cause of Dementia in the world. This cognitive loss hampers your reasoning, remembering thinking and other behavioural traits, affecting your day-to-day routines.
3. **Huntington's**: This is a rare hereditary neurological disease caused by mutation of genes leading to progressive breakdown. Brain damage is caused by collection of toxic proteins in the brains. This critically impacts functionality of a person resulting in loss of thinking, movement and at times leading to psychiatric disorders. Huntington's symptoms usually occur at the age of thirty or forty and sometimes rarely in the age of twenty also, known as juvenile Huntington cases. Medications can help patients but can't prevent decline in behavioural, mental, and physical conditions in patients.
4. **MS or Multiple Sclerosis**: MS is an unpredictable disease hampering the central nervous system, thus critically impacting the optic nerves, spinal cord, and the brain at large. This interrupts the smooth flow of information between mind and body. This NDDs is most common disabling medical concern in young adults between twenty and forty. Myelin in the central nervous system is mistakenly attacked by the immune system cells leading to loss of protection from unhealthy cells, bacteria and other harmful viruses seriously impacting the total nervous system. The disease is a chronic disease and not fatal, affecting different people differently.
5. **ALS or Amyotrophic Lateral Sclerosis**: ALS a motor neuron disorder is also known as the Lou Gehrig disease affecting the nerves that control your muscles. This gets worse over time and is progressive. The loss of voluntary muscles impacts your vital actions like movements of arms and legs, speaking, breathing,

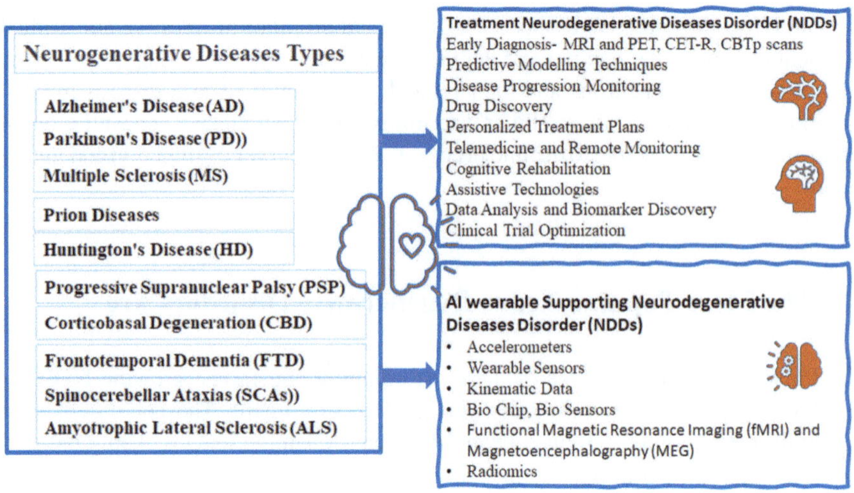

Fig. 3 NDDs and treatment

and eating, often leading to paralysis. There is a positive improvement in the treatment procedures of ALS patients, corrective medical measures can slow-down the progression of the disease and improve the quality of patient's life. This in non-hereditary, where in 90% cases have no gene mutation or family history involved.

Till date the root causes of neurodegenerative diseases are not completely understandable, but they are thought to be derived from composite and complex interplay of lifestyle, environmental and genetic integrations. Presently there is no fully curable treatments of neurodegenerative diseases and there are fewer treatment and medicinal options for this complex progressive disease. But the future looks hopeful with progressive medicinal gains in the fields of neuroscience, drugs and genetics with digital amalgamations spearheading the novel diagnostics, treatments, and therapies. Research and Development in Neurodegenerative diseases field is going on at a herculean pace aimed to better understand the progressive ailment. counter it with new progressive treatments, therapies, and medicine in which Artificial Intelligence is leading from the front integrating digital systems (Fig. 3).

5 Recent Research and Development in Neuro Degenerative Disorders Field Are

1. **Artificial Intelligence**: AI through advanced communication and digital acoustics is analysing huge data sets, medical images, genomic data & biomarkers to identify, analyse and predict the diseases and its patterns. This helps in personal

patient diagnosis and faster treatment. AI visualizes and predicts how medicines, machines and drugs will act in the patient's body; it also proactively provides personal treatment by controlling machine enabled drug delivery systems to administer drugs in measured environments.

2. **Stem Cell Therapy**: In last more than two decades stem cell therapies have enabled positive results in new age treatments and investigations of NDDs. Stem cells can develop diverse types of cells & tissues and can act as repair and rebuild mechanisms for the body. Adult stem cells and Embryonic stem cells are the two main type of stem cells. These are mainly harvested from peripheral blood and bone marrow. With their conversion, regeneration, and proliferation ability to mark and enable undifferentiated cells and tissues to production of differentiated ones, makes them unique and a match winner. Cellular therapies are widely popular options of treatment in NDDs, and stem cell research is widely being pursued in the medicinal treatment field.
3. **Genetics**: The root causes of NDDs are varied but genetics signify many neurodegenerative cases and thus it becomes even more mandatory area of genetic research to evaluate patients with ASD, GDD &ID. Genetic diagnosis and investigation is strongly prescribed for affected patients. Evidence based treatments like descriptive & genetic evaluation and diagnosis help affected families become familiar and acclimatize with the medical conditions prevailing and for prognosis and recurrence detection. The demand for genetic counsellors increases manifold to handle the huge demand of genetic evaluations as they sympathetically counsel, guide and educate the families on the diverse modes of test and treatments being offered to the patient.
4. **Biomarkers**: These new age technologies are providing robust, cost effective and objective based NDD treatment in the medical fields. Psychology, behavioural enhancement, and development in motor functionality can help in correct analysis of neo degenerative condition and degradation. There are four types of biomarkers Histologic, Molecular, Radiographic and Physiologic. Medicinal fraternity finds a growing need for efficient biomarkers to enable practical and research based NDDs functioning. This will help in clear diagnosis, monitored recovery, smooth rehabilitation, and help in correct projections. These digital cognitive and behavioural bio markers are redefining medical approaches to neuro disabilities. There is a higher demand of researching and developing novel imaging biomarkers for NDDs for therapeutic personal patient care [19]. Biomarkers should be enabled by new neuroimaging techniques which are most perfect to integrate due to its cost effectiveness, extensive distribution, non-invasiveness and its capacity to outline the functioning and formation structure of the brain.

Development of Drugs: Drug Development is a costly, time consuming and intricate process and it's the same for neurodegenerative diseases. NDD drug development needs basket trials with precise optimization which should be strictly as per compliance from FDA and other medical regulatory agencies. This will reduce redundancies in the trial processes, strengthen implementation, increase awareness, enable more recruitments, identifying relevant biomarkers, coordination of placebo groups and integration in clinical trials for the treatment of neurodegenerative diseases. There is an imminent need to quickly research on new drugs, molecular targets, varied screening systems and path mechanisms, also identifying new tracks, new therapeutics, innovative formyl peptide receptors, effect of natural anti-inflammatory composites & fungal byproducts.

Lifestyle Routines: As per medical experts, your fitness and daily routine regimes should be upright to reduce the risk of neurodegenerative diseases. Focus on diet, exercise, healthy lifestyle, alert mental health is critical for keeping safe distance from neurodegenerative diseases [22]. Physical exercise is a general strategy to keep medical problems away by being fit and healthy. This keeps your cardio, respiratory, blood pressure and metabolic levels under control and improves your cognitive functions. Apart from being an effective medical approach, it enhances the body by increasing stamina, endurance, muscles, blood circulation, motor skills, muscles, elasticity, mobility, oxygen level intake and reflexes which is vital for brain and body functioning [9]. A healthy lifestyle reduces stress levels, anxiety and detoxification against unhealthy food and severity of pathologies. Meditation, yoga, and physiotherapies are advised by doctors to patients in progressive diseases also to improve the body mind balance which is a vital aspect in NDDs. Physical & Sports therapies and treatments also provide hope and improvement in the life of neuro patients and are very effective in improving their daily lifestyles. However, there is an imminent need to constantly understand, research and develop new, cost effective and personalized treatments for such critical medical cases.

6 Critical Role of AI in Enabling Smooth Medical Progressions for Neurodegenerative Treatments

Natural Language Processing: By analysing huge data sets including scientific literature, medicinal records, research pedagogies, patients case histories, AI processes the data with algorithmic integrations to predict patterns and foresights to be used in neurodegenerative treatments.

Medical imaging analysis: AI algorithms are being developed to analyse medical imaging data such as MRI and PET scans to identify early signs of neurodegenerative diseases. For example, AI can detect changes in brain structure and function that may indicate Alzheimer's disease before symptoms appear.

Genomic analysis: AI is being used to analyse large datasets of genomic data to identify genetic factors that contribute to the development of neurodegenerative diseases. This information can be used to develop personalized treatments and interventions.

Drug discovery: AI is being used to identify new drug targets and develop new treatments for neurodegenerative diseases. For example, AI can predict how specific drugs will interact with target proteins and identify potential side effects.

Personalized medicine: AI is being used to develop personalized treatment plans based on an individual's unique genetic and clinical profile. This approach could lead to more effective treatments with fewer side effects.

Overall, AI has the potential to revolutionize our understanding of neurodegenerative diseases by analysing vast amounts of data and identifying patterns and insights that may be missed by traditional methods. However, much work remains to be done to fully realize the potential of AI in this field.

Cases where AI is enabling smooth medical transitions of neurodegenerative diseases.

Virtual Assistants: In Alzheimer's and other neurodegenerative diseases like dementia, AI aided virtual assistants are proving the turning point in helping the progressive disease medical patients. The popular virtual assistants like Telemedicine, Telehealth, Personal ALS Voice Assistant, Louise, Virtual Physical Therapy Assistant, Avecen, Voice Based Diet Assistant, Google Home & Amazon are using voice and easy manual digital commands to enable patients or their helpers to aid in therapies and medicinal support. Virtual Assistants are like true companions and helping in many essential days to day tasks such as, setting reminders, playing music through voice commands, and answering to medicinal, health and general queries. Various research and studies conducted to evaluate the performance of virtual assistants in NDDs have proved them to be an asset in treatment of neuro patients. They have enhanced the mind, quality of life and temperament of patients as they are helping them being independent again. By being their friendly communicative companion, they have helped in making them more independent, determined and feel less lonely. They are proving to be a real boon for the patient's family and their helpers too.

Wearable Devices: Artificial Intelligence driven wearable devices are proving to be an asset in fight against NDDs as they are timely and accurately measuring and tracking neuro patients' progressions and charting future course of actions and tests in accordance with medical experts [20]. In Parkinson's, Alzheimer's and other neuro disorders these devices have correctly detected abnormal symptoms and shocks in patients' body to be tended by doctors in accordance with treatment required [10]. These wearable devices have proved to be consistent, precise, and well adaptable to patients. ICT, Wearable Accelerometers, CT-Radiomics, Wearable Sensors, Kinematic Data. These wearable digital devices are enabling patients and their families with vital medical communications by identifying problems remotely. They can be easily mapped with our daily routines and have been incorporated in mobiles, apps, watches, glasses, caps, shoes, shirts, bracelets, rings etc. AI enabled wearable market is expected to touch $ 70 billion by 2026. Timely monitorization and analyzation of patient's health through reports and data help the doctors and family distantly also by acting as lifesaving agents in critical conditions like pre detecting seizures and other brain and heart attacks.

Neuro Degenerative Disorders AI Forecasting & Diagnostics Tools: AI has made breathtaking breakthroughs in early predictions and accurate diagnosis for neurology disorders. The use of tools like Bio Chips and Bio Sensors are enabling

Vitro diagnostics. AI uses Micro Array data through Machine Learning integrations to interpret, classify and perceive the abnormalities in patients. Neuro Imaging helps in understanding the functions of the brain. Structural Imaging & Functional Imaging helps decode brain structure and functioning. Functional MRI (FMRI) outlines the key areas of activations in the brain by comparing, tracking, evaluating, and mapping the brain activities and respondent's pace. Megnetoencephalography (MEG) scan identifies and measures the magnetic fields in the brain and brain Position Emission Tomography (PET) scan helps in brain imaging. Radiomics is effectively assisting radiologist in neuro oncology by predicting the infiltrating margins of progression, recurrence, and survival in neuro diseases. Gadolinium MRI detects glioblastoma cancer in the brain and spine by evaluating perfusion and diffusion in the patient's body. Further AI aided spectroscopy and histopathology helps to diagnose the inbuilt characteristics of glioblastoma, helping in predicting recurrences and therapeutic responses post treatment. Through radioactive tracer it evaluates any injury or diseases in the brain. These tools can transform healthcare by their ability to predict the medical discrepancies early and accurately in the brain and body, thus enabling personalized treatments.

There are many more AI enabled technologies that are proving to be game changers in the fight against NDDs. The support, personalised care, medical services and monitoring they provide are second to none and a boon for the patient and their families. No doubt there is ample scope to improve on these technologies being more relevant and in sync with the medical problems. There is also an imminent need to make these devices more affordable, accessible, and easy to use for the patients. Virtual Assistants and Wearable Devices are helping patients in constantly updating, self-management, enhancing medical routines, being cautious and regularly accessing and judging the health, behaviour and upholding the value of life by adhering to the best practices in case of Neuro Patients.

7 Potential AI Risks Including Medical Fields

Though AI grows at a stupendous pace with its advanced miraculous digital technology and smart communication systems it finds itself surrounded by potential dangers and murky waters. It is an accepted game changing machine learning revolution with certain drawbacks to be measured, countered, and worked upon [24].

Violating Privacy: Regulations and compliance is vital to AI technology and its advance systems as it also enhances security and privacy risks in healthcare industry [21]. With its huge possibility to bring in sweeping changes in clinical research, diagnosis, and care delivery. AI collects data of patients while interacting, but it's vital to know its end use. This collected personal data or user experience customization data banks are further used in diverse AI Models to predict outcomes. Data privacy tools should be foolproof against any data theft, data sale, data sharing or hacking attacks. Cyber laws should be made strong and stringent against all digital interfaces and its facilitators.

Lacking in Explainability & Transparency: The deep learning models are intricate and tough to understand even for engineers and scientists involved in making or using them. It makes it more elusive and mysterious as to how AI comes to a particular answer and conclusions. So, this creates a mystery on the use of data algorithms by AI and there is no further clarity on it making unsafe or biased outcomes. This has made explainable AI more popular but still lots of work must be done on transparencies. Patients will get further confused and helpless, if they are not able to understand the digitalised systems, process, and outcomes.

Manipulating Social Platforms: Social platforms can be used aggressively to manipulate mindsets through AI. This can leave positive and negative impacts in the society. AI enables Twitter, Facebook, LinkedIn, Instagram for content moderation, data analysis and info graphics. With collection of sensitive data of users like preferences, likes and time spent, it can help advertisers and companies manipulate mindsets in accordance. News and Media has been affected by AI enabled fake videos and images, lip syncing, bogus content, swapping data, manipulations through voice changers, video hoaxes and deep fakes have instigated thefts and hacking of data [12]. Personal data and privacy of patients in such critical medical scenario is critical information and manipulation on media platforms can dither their confidentiality.

Job Security: With spurge in digital automation in systems and devices by AI, there will be job losses and manpower restrictions in manufacturing, healthcare, sales, and marketing. AI automation will trigger low unemployment rate as robots and chatbots will require fewer human interventions. These machines and systems will require human interfaces, an intelligent balance between man and machine can be an ideal scenario for the job service sector. Upskilling for technical support is vital for survival in the ever-changing technology world. Though AI will displace the job sector, but it will also create numerous new technical jobs in the medical and other sectors.

Social Scrutiny: Security and privacy are critical threats in medical industry as well; some countries & companies are using AI technologies for monitoring staff at workplaces. It becomes problematic when you breach the trust from official hours to personal monitorisation. Also, when being used in surveillance by legal authorities it can lead to biases as AI algorithms are not foolproof and can misjudge identities [2]. Deepfakes in AI are also of a critical concern for personal and organizational security as they can mask and manipulate data, identity and crucial information leading to decremental health of the concerned. One person's identity can be covered and clearly swapped with another for various gains. Here content is portrayed to be authenticated by your known or well-acquainted figures to repose faith in the wrongly scripted agenda or forged tactics. Many such examples have been depicted in elections, war, product launches and even major corporate board decisions, which when thoroughly investigated were found to be manipulated or forged.

Biases: Technology is taking the bias scenarios beyond race, sex, power, wealth, and gender by showing unpredictive discrepancies in algorithms and databases [13]. We can say its human nature to take sides as per convenience and AI also is human's imagination and invention. This in technical term is also known as Algorithm bias, AI bias or Machine Learning bias. Bias propagates discrimination and encourages mistrust among people hampering their mindsets. Bias among patients can be critical and can cause huge mistrust among their families. AI scientists and engineers must ensure that new systems, their research, and standards improve human decision making them foolproof to reduce their flaws and bias interventions.

Economic Disparity: Socio economic disparities are highlighted by AI's intricate and unexplainable algorithms. This compromises the Diversity, Equity, and Inclusion (DEI) philosophy as AI tends to analyse candidate's personality and traits through his voice and face, feature analysation. Also, AI reflects on job performances by poorly categorising repetitive job workers in one category and excluding or ignoring higher level job employees. All HR departments including medical sector are advised to abstain from such discriminatory hiring practices.

Compromising Goodwill & Ethics: AI somewhere compromises on value systems and effects the socio-economic fabric structure. At times incorrect data and biased opinions is propagated and circulated by AI to form opinions which can be overbearing, even in the medical field. Technology is very important but technological prowess should not overpower human goodwill.

Judicious use of Autonomous Systems & Mechanisms: Digitalised revolutions should not get into adverse hands to be misused against mankind. Robotics should enable humanity and not fuel enmity and destruction. AI has the power to be moulded both ways, humans must control it wisely for development and best end use. It can be used as a growth supplement or blessing or a potent and complex mechanism. Developers must be constantly wary of malicious and infiltrating agents and plan their risk mitigation strategies in accordance.

Economic upheaval: Economic markets are using AI in trading and various financial transactions and any flaw in algorithmic trading may cause imminent turmoil. This can trigger mistrust, fear and collapse of markets and economies in general. Set patterns at blazing pace can lead to chain reactions and sudden volatility across all industries adversely affecting economic and physical health. AI are also helping people to be more learned and market smart.

Loosing Human Touch: Digital technology distances the human touch as machines at times tend to overpower human interactions. Using AI in healthcare diminishes human touch, empathy, creativity, reasoning, and emotional expression. Too much dependency on digital machines will tend to reduce social skills and peer interactions.

Overpowering Control: Loosing human touch is the biggest fear for AI. Technology should never go beyond human control. It should be creative and not destructive. Imitating self and others for negative propositions can lead to grave destructions and disruptions. Machine Learning researchers must curb these negative aspirations and enhance technological advancement to augment humanity.

8 Conclusion

AI through Machine Learning integrations and Neural Networks can inspire human minds towards research and analysis to produce problem solving measures in human ecology [11]. Precision medicine backed by smart communication systems and power data banks of Artificial Intelligence are essential for treatment against Neurodegenerative progressive disease [23]. We must move ahead to effective and innovative inclusive medical approach and prefer personal diagnosis and treatment, from prior approach of one size fitting for all. With advancements in AI and machine learning systems, algorithmics are developed with deep learning and researching huge pool of data banks which are providing frameworks for more precise diagnosis and therapeutic approaches. These tools are being helpful in generating the responses of present treatments and evaluating the risk of further disease progressions. Imaging Techniques, Biomarkers, MRI, CT & Radiomics for prognosis and treatment are vital in mapping these progressive neuro ailments. Thus, AI backed predictive forecasting analysis mapped with NDDs diagnostic evaluation and detailed heredity health status are proving a comprehensive risk mitigation tool in fight against these critical neuro ailments [8]. The whole world positively expects AI backed digital systems to counter and curb the substantial burden that neurodegenerative diseases are imposing on the medical fraternity, neuro patients and their families [18]. Early diagnosis, best prevention and cost effective and comprehensive treatment are more than expected from AI novel technologies and they're being the turning point against the devastating NDD diseases affecting millions globally.

References

1. Alyssa Blesson, J. S. (2019). Genetic counseling in neurodevelopmental disorders. *Cold Spring Horbor*.
2. Barney, N. (n.d.). *deepfake AI (deep fake)*. Retrieved from www.techtarget.com: https://www.techtarget.com/whatis/definition/deepfake.
3. Beck, A. T. (2019). *What is recovery-oriented cognitive therapy (CT-R)?* Retrieved from www.beckinstitute.org: https://beckinstitute.org/blog/what-is-recovery-oriented-cognitive-therapy-ct-r/.
4. Behor, N. (2021). *Linkedin*. Retrieved from What is Wearable AI And How it Can Change the World?: https://www.linkedin.com/pulse/what-wearable-ai-how-can-change-world-nil-behor/.
5. Bi, C., Zhou, S., Liu, X., Zhu, Y., Yu, J., Zhang, X., Shi, M., Wu, R., He, H., Zhan, C., Lin, Y., & Shen, B. (2022). NDDRF: A risk factor knowledgebase for personalized prevention of neurodegenerative diseases. *Journal of Advanced Research, 40*, 223–231.https://doi.org/10.1016/j.jare.2021.06.015
6. Dhivya Venkatesan, A. E. (2022). *Diagnostic and therapeutic approach of artificial intelligence in neuro-oncological diseases*. Elsevier.
7. Dong, L., Yang, Q., Zhang, R. H., & Wei, W. B. (2021). Artificial intelligence for the detection of age-related macular degeneration in color fundus photographs: A systematic review and meta-analysis. *EClinicalMedicine, 35*, 100875. https://doi.org/10.1016/j.eclinm.2021.100875

8. Ellis, M. (2018). *How artificial intelligence is tackling neurodegerenrative diseases.* Retrieved from https://www.proclinical.com/: https://www.proclinical.com/blogs/2018-4/how-ai-is-tackling-neurodegenerative-diseases
9. Elodie Kip, L. C.-B. (2023). Healthy lifestyles and wellbeing reduce neuroinflammation and prevent neurodegenerative and psychiatric disorders. *Frontiers.*
10. Guillermo Prieto -Avalos, L. N.-M. (2022). A review of commercial and non-commercial wearables devices for monitoring motor impairments caused by neurodegenerative diseases. *National Library of Medicine.*
11. Guoguang Wong, A. M. (2020). Artificial intelligence in healthcare: Review and prediction case studies. *Elsevier.*
12. Harwell, D. (2019). An artificial-intelligence first: Voice-mimicking software reportedly used in a major theft. *The Washington Post.*
13. James Manyika, J. S. (2019). What do we do about the biases in AI? *Howard Business Review.*
14. Julie, C., & Chow, F. H. (2023). *Prediction of neurodevelopmental disorders based on de novo coding variation. Springer.*
15. Kepp, K. P. (2019). A quantitative model of human neurodegenerative diseases involving protein aggregation. Neurobiol. Aging 80, *Kepp, K. P. (2019). A quantitative model of human neurodegenerati.* https://doi.org/10.1016/j.neurobiolaging.2019.04.001, 46–55.
16. Kumar, A. V., Kumar, S., Garg, V. K., Goel, N., Hoang, V. T., & Kashyap, D. (2023). Future perspectives for automated neurodegenerative disorders diagnosis: Challenges and possible research directions. *Springer, Singapore.* https://doi.org/10.1007/978-981-99-2154-6_15
17. Kwon, D. (2022). Scientific American Article "Eye Tests May Help Diagnose Alzheimer's Disease. *Springer Nature.* Retrieved September Friday, 2023, from https://www.scientificamerican.com/article/eye-tests-may-help-diagnose-alzheimer-rsquo-s-disease
18. Maria J., & Molnar, V. M. (2023). AI-based tools for the diagnosis and treatment of rare neurological disorders. *Nature Reviews.*
19. Mark Crook Rumsey, S. J. (2023). Multicohort cross-sectional study of cognitive and behavioural digital biomarkers in neurodegeneration. *BMJ.*
20. Mattia Franchi de Cavalieri, S. F. (2023). Wearable accelerometers for measuring and monitoring the motor behaviour of infants with brain damage during CareToy-Revised training. *Journal of Neuro Engineering and Rehabilitation .*
21. Mckeon, J. (n.d.). *Security, Privacy Risks of Artificial Intelligence in Healthcare.* Retrieved from www.healthisecurity.com: https://healthitsecurity.com/features/security-privacy-risks-of-artificial-intelligence-in-healthcare
22. Roberto Bonanni, I. C. (2022). Physical exercise and health: A focus on its protective role in neurodegenerative diseases. *Functional Morphology and Kinesiology.*
23. Sharyn, L., & Rossi, P. S. (2023). The future is precision medicine-guided diagnoses, preventions and treatments for neurodegenerative diseases. *Frontiers.*
24. Thomas, M. (2023). *12 Risks and Dangers of Artificial Intelligence (AI).* Retrieved from www.builtin.com: https://builtin.com/artificial-intelligence/risks-of-artificial-intelligence
25. Wongi Seoul, H. K. (2020). Urinary biomarkers for neurodegenerative diseases. *Researchgate.*

Ethical Considerations: Case Scenarios

Loveleen Gaur and Devanshi Gaur

Abstract The integration of eXplainable Artificial Intelligence (XAI) in the management of neurodegenerative diseases presents immense potential for improved patient care and medical research. However, it also raises profound ethical considerations that must be meticulously addressed. The chapter will highlight case scenarios which demonstrate the importance of addressing ethical considerations when implementing XAI in the context of neurodegenerative diseases. It is essential to develop guidelines, standards, and governance structures that promote responsible and ethical AI use while maximizing the benefits of these technologies in improving patient care.

Keywords Explainable artificial intelligence · Neurodegenerative diseases · Advancements in neuroimaging

1 Introduction

XAI holds immense promise in enhancing neurodegenerative disease management, ethical considerations are pivotal to ensure that patient rights, privacy, and values are upheld, and that the technology ultimately benefits both patients and healthcare providers. The integration of eXplainable Artificial Intelligence (XAI) in the management of neurodegenerative diseases presents immense potential for improved patient care and medical research. However, it also raises profound ethical considerations that must be meticulously addressed [1, 2].

Data privacy emerges as a paramount concern. Patient data in neurodegenerative diseases often includes highly sensitive medical records, genetic information, and real-time monitoring data. Protecting this information is essential to preserve patient confidentiality and uphold their rights. Robust encryption, secure storage, and strict

L. Gaur (✉)
Taylor's University, Subang Jaya, Malaysia
e-mail: gaurloveleen@yahoo.com

D. Gaur
Florida International University, Miami, USA

© The Author(s), under exclusive license to Springer Nature Switzerland AG 2024
L. Gaur et al. (eds.), *AI and Neuro-Degenerative Diseases*, Studies in Computational Intelligence 1131, https://doi.org/10.1007/978-3-031-53148-4_10

access controls are indispensable safeguards. Furthermore, the informed consent of patients, where they fully understand and willingly agree to the use of their data, is imperative in research and clinical applications.

Transparency and interpretability of AI recommendations are pivotal ethical factors. It is essential that healthcare providers and patients can comprehend the rationale behind AI-driven decisions. Transparent insights instill trust in the AI system, enabling more confident decision-making.

Addressing algorithmic bias and ensuring fairness is vital to prevent discrimination in healthcare. AI models must be rigorously tested for biases and corrected to deliver equitable recommendations across diverse patient demographics.

Respecting patient autonomy and involvement is another ethical cornerstone. AI should augment, not supplant, healthcare decisions. Patients must have the final say in their treatment plans, with AI serving as an aid that aligns with their values and preferences.

Human oversight and accountability remain crucial. While AI contributes to healthcare, healthcare providers ultimately shoulder the responsibility for patient outcomes. Robust accountability mechanisms must be in place to rectify errors or adverse events involving AI [3–5].

Ethical review boards, regulatory compliance, long-term monitoring, and interdisciplinary collaboration are additional ethical considerations that together ensure the responsible and ethical integration of XAI in the realm of neurodegenerative diseases.

2 Key Areas

Ethical considerations surrounding the use of eXplainable Artificial Intelligence (XAI) in the context of neurodegenerative diseases are paramount. These considerations encompass several key areas:

- *Patient Data Privacy*: Protecting the privacy and security of patient data, which often includes sensitive medical records, genetic information, and real-time monitoring data, is essential. Ethical use of XAI requires robust data encryption, secure storage, and strict access controls. Informed consent from patients for data usage in research and clinical applications is also crucial.
- *Transparency and Interpretability*: XAI models must provide clear and understandable explanations for their decisions. Ensuring that healthcare providers and patients can comprehend and trust the AI-driven recommendations is fundamental for ethical AI use. Transparent insights maintain trust in the AI system.
- *Algorithm Bias and Fairness*: Developers and healthcare institutions must address biases in AI models. Detecting and mitigating bias ensures that AI recommendations do not lead to discriminatory outcomes. Ethical AI strives for fairness, delivering consistent and unbiased recommendations across different patient demographics.

- *Patient Autonomy and Involvement*: Patient autonomy in healthcare decisions should be upheld. While AI can provide valuable insights, the final decision-making authority must rest with the patient. Patients should have access to understandable explanations of AI's impact on their diagnosis, treatment, and care.
- *Oversight and Accountability*: Human oversight remains essential in healthcare. Healthcare providers are ultimately accountable for patient outcomes, and AI should assist them rather than replace their judgment. Accountability mechanisms should be in place to address errors or adverse events involving AI.
- *Ethical Review and Regulatory Compliance*: Independent ethical review boards should evaluate the use of AI and XAI in healthcare settings to ensure adherence to ethical standards. Compliance with healthcare regulations and data protection laws is essential to safeguard patient rights and data security.
- *Long-Term Monitoring and Impact Assessment*: Ethical considerations extend beyond initial AI implementation. The long-term impact of AI on patient outcomes and healthcare delivery should be continually monitored and assessed. AI systems should adapt to evolving ethical and medical guidelines.
- *Collaboration and Interdisciplinary Ethics*: Ethical AI implementation requires collaboration between AI developers, healthcare professionals, regulatory bodies, and patients themselves. An interdisciplinary approach ensures that ethical considerations are addressed comprehensively.

In summary, ethical considerations in the use of XAI in neurodegenerative diseases revolve around data privacy, transparency, fairness, patient autonomy, oversight, compliance, long-term impact, and collaborative ethics. Upholding these ethical principles is essential to ensure that AI technologies contribute to improved patient care while respecting individual rights and values [6–8].

3 Case Scenarios

The ethical challenges in the application of XAI in healthcare can be illustrated by general examples that apply to neurodegenerative diseases as well. Here are a few potential scenarios that highlight ethical considerations:

Case Scenario 1: Patient Data Privacy

A prominent research institution embarks on an ambitious project to develop an eXplainable Artificial Intelligence (XAI) model aimed at predicting the disease progression of patients afflicted with neurodegenerative diseases. The objective is to harness the power of AI to provide healthcare providers with valuable insights that can aid in personalized treatment plans and early interventions. However, the development and deployment of this XAI model presents a set of intricate ethical considerations.

Data Collection and Utilization: The research institution begins by assembling a comprehensive dataset. This dataset includes a wide array of information, such as the patients' medical records, genetic profiles, and real-time data gathered from wearable devices. These sources of data offer a multifaceted view of each patient's health status, progression, and responses to treatments [9, 10].

Ethical Considerations:

- *Patient Data Privacy*: The inclusion of sensitive patient information in the dataset necessitates stringent measures to safeguard data privacy. This involves employing state-of-the-art encryption techniques to protect data both in transit and at rest. Additionally, robust access controls ensure that only authorized personnel can access and utilize this sensitive data.
- *Informed Consent*: Respecting patient autonomy and informed decision-making is paramount. Patients must be provided with clear and comprehensive information about how their data will be used in this research endeavor. Obtaining informed consent ensures that individuals willingly and knowingly agree to participate in the study.
- *Transparency and Interpretability*: As the XAI model is designed to provide explainable insights, efforts are made to ensure that the predictions and recommendations generated by the model are transparent and interpretable. This transparency fosters trust among healthcare providers, patients, and their families.
- *Data Security*: Beyond encryption, secure storage facilities are employed to prevent unauthorized access or data breaches. Stringent cybersecurity protocols are implemented to mitigate the risk of cyberattacks that could compromise patient data.
- *Fairness and Bias Mitigation*: The research institution rigorously assesses the XAI model for biases. Steps are taken to ensure that the model's predictions are unbiased and do not discriminate against any particular patient demographic. Fairness is a guiding principle in the development process.
- *Patient Involvement*: Throughout the project, patients are actively engaged and kept informed about the progress. Their feedback and perspectives are valued, and their right to be involved in decisions regarding their healthcare data is respected.
- *Oversight and Accountability*: Ethical oversight is maintained through the involvement of independent ethical review boards. Additionally, mechanisms for accountability are established to address any issues or discrepancies that may arise during the development and deployment of the XAI model.

In essence, this case scenario underscores the intricate ethical considerations that accompany the development of XAI models for predicting disease progression in neurodegenerative diseases. Balancing the potential benefits of AI-driven insights with the ethical imperatives of data privacy, transparency, fairness, and patient autonomy is essential to ensure responsible and ethical research practices [11–14].

Case Scenario 2: Transparency and Trust

Within the halls of a modern hospital, a cutting-edge initiative unfolds as healthcare professionals deploy an eXplainable Artificial Intelligence (XAI) decision support system. This system is specifically designed to provide invaluable assistance to clinicians in the challenging task of diagnosing neurodegenerative diseases. However, a profound ethical and operational challenge emerges as the system's output is unveiled—it is a complex black-box model, shrouded in a veil of opacity. The clinicians, despite their expertise and experience, grapple with a perplexing predicament: comprehending how this AI-driven system arrives at its diagnostic recommendations [15–18].

Complexity Amid Potential: The XAI-powered decision support system represents a technological marvel, capable of processing vast troves of patient data, including medical records, imaging scans, genetic profiles, and real-time sensor data. It harnesses the power of advanced machine learning algorithms to analyze this data and generate diagnostic recommendations. While the potential of such a system is immense, its complexity raises profound questions.

Ethical Considerations:

- *Transparency Imperative*: The lack of transparency within the black-box model becomes an ethical focal point. Healthcare providers are confronted with the challenge of understanding the inner workings of the AI system. The ethical imperative here is to ensure that AI-generated recommendations are transparent and interpretable.
- *Clinician Trust*: Trust is fundamental in healthcare decision-making. Clinicians, who bear the responsibility for patient care, must have confidence in the AI-driven recommendations. Ethical considerations dictate that AI systems must provide clinicians with insights they can trust to make informed decisions.
- *Patient Outcomes*: At the core of this scenario is the ethical obligation to prioritize patient outcomes. Timely and accurate diagnoses are critical in neurodegenerative diseases. If clinicians cannot fully comprehend the AI recommendations, it may impact patient care and potentially delay essential treatments.
- *Collaborative Care*: Ethical healthcare revolves around a collaborative approach. While AI can be a powerful tool, it should enhance, not replace, the expertise of healthcare providers. The challenge is to strike the right balance between AI-driven insights and the clinical acumen of the care team.
- *Interdisciplinary Ethical Review*: To navigate this complex scenario ethically, interdisciplinary teams and ethical review boards play a pivotal role. Their involvement ensures that the AI system aligns with ethical principles while maximizing its potential benefits [19, 20].

The deployment of an XAI-driven decision support system in the diagnosis of neurodegenerative diseases presents both promise and complexity. Ethical considerations demand a commitment to transparency, trust, patient outcomes, collaborative care, and rigorous ethical oversight. The journey toward harnessing AI's potential while upholding ethical standards is a dynamic and evolving one, shaping the future of healthcare.

Case Scenario 3: Algorithm Bias and Fairness

Within the realm of diagnosing neurodegenerative diseases, an advanced eXplainable Artificial Intelligence (XAI) model stands at the forefront of medical innovation. This model, designed to aid in the diagnostic process, appears to hold immense potential. However, an ethical quandary surfaces as a concerning pattern becomes evident—the XAI model exhibits bias in its diagnostic recommendations. Specifically, these biases manifest in a manner that leads to delayed or incorrect diagnoses, disproportionately affecting certain demographic groups [21, 22].

The Promise and the Predicament: The XAI model in question represents a leap forward in healthcare, harnessing the power of machine learning and data analysis to assist healthcare providers in diagnosing neurodegenerative diseases. It draws upon extensive datasets comprising patient records, imaging scans, and genetic information to generate recommendations. Yet, the revelation of bias within this model raises profound ethical considerations.

Ethical Implications:

- *Bias Detection and Mitigation*: The foremost ethical imperative revolves around the detection and mitigation of bias. It is incumbent upon healthcare institutions and AI developers to identify and rectify any prejudiced patterns in the XAI model. Addressing bias is crucial to ensure equitable and fair healthcare delivery.
- *Equity in Healthcare*: The ethical cornerstone here is equity. AI systems in healthcare should provide consistent and unbiased recommendations to all patient groups, regardless of demographics. The disproportionate impact on specific populations calls for a reevaluation of model training and data sources.
- *Patient Well-Being*: The overarching ethical concern is the well-being of patients. Delayed or incorrect diagnoses in neurodegenerative diseases can have severe consequences for individuals' health and quality of life. Ethical healthcare dictates that AI models prioritize accurate and timely diagnoses for all patients.
- *Transparency and Accountability*: Ethical AI demands transparency in both the development and deployment of models. Healthcare providers and patients should be informed about the presence of bias and how it is being addressed. Furthermore, mechanisms for accountability should be established to address any adverse effects stemming from biased recommendations.
- *Continuous Evaluation*: The ethical journey does not end with bias mitigation. Continuous evaluation and monitoring of AI systems are imperative. Regular assessments for fairness and bias should be integrated into the model's lifecycle to ensure ongoing ethical AI practice.

The scenario underscores the ethical challenges associated with bias in AI-driven diagnosis of neurodegenerative diseases. The ethical path forward calls for vigilance, transparency, equity, and a commitment to patient well-being. As AI continues to shape the landscape of healthcare, addressing bias becomes not only an ethical obligation but also a critical step in delivering just, accurate, and equitable care to all [23].

Case Scenario 4: Patient Autonomy

In the realm of healthcare for neurodegenerative diseases, an innovative eXplainable Artificial Intelligence (XAI)-based decision support system takes center stage. This system, designed to provide treatment recommendations, holds the promise of improving patient care. However, an ethical quandary unfolds when it becomes evident that the system's recommendations fail to align with a patient's deeply held personal preferences and values [24].

The Promise and the Ethical Dilemma: The XAI-based decision support system is engineered to assist patients suffering from neurodegenerative diseases. It leverages advanced algorithms to analyze patient data, clinical records, and research findings, culminating in personalized treatment recommendations. Despite its potential to enhance care, the ethical dimension emerges as the system's recommendations often diverge from the patient's individual preferences and values.

Ethical Considerations:

- *Patient-Centric Care*: At the heart of healthcare ethics lies patient-centric care. The ethical imperative here is to prioritize the patient's autonomy and values. AI systems should align their recommendations with what matters most to the patient, ensuring that treatment plans resonate with their preferences.
- *Informed Decision-Making*: Ethical healthcare upholds the principle of informed decision-making. Patients must be well-informed about their treatment options and understand the implications of each choice. If the XAI recommendations deviate from a patient's values, it is essential to communicate this misalignment transparently.
- *Shared Decision-Making*: Collaboration between patients and healthcare providers is pivotal. Ethical practice dictates that treatment decisions should be made jointly, considering the patient's desires, concerns, and the clinical expertise of the healthcare team. AI should facilitate this collaborative approach rather than override patient values.
- *Patient Empowerment*: Ethical AI empowers patients. It provides them with the tools and knowledge necessary to actively participate in their healthcare decisions. Patients have the right to voice their preferences and values, and the AI system should adapt to accommodate these individual perspectives.
- *Ethical Oversight*: To navigate this ethical challenge, healthcare institutions should establish ethical oversight mechanisms. These mechanisms ensure that AI systems respect patient values, promote shared decision-making, and prioritize patient autonomy.

The scenario highlights the ethical complexities that can arise when XAI-based decision support systems intersect with deeply personal patient values. Ethical healthcare demands that AI systems not only provide recommendations but also ensure that these recommendations align with the patient's unique preferences and values. The ethical path forward involves recognizing and respecting individual autonomy while leveraging AI to enhance the quality of care in neurodegenerative diseases.

Case Scenario 5: Oversight and Accountability

Within the realm of neurodegenerative disease management, a healthcare provider embarks on an ambitious initiative, placing considerable reliance on an advanced eXplainable Artificial Intelligence (XAI) system. This system assumes a pivotal role in making treatment decisions for patients grappling with these challenging conditions. However, a pressing ethical dilemma arises as the system's recommendations, in certain instances, lead to adverse outcomes for patients [25].

The Promise and the Ethical Challenge: The XAI system represents a beacon of hope in the complex landscape of neurodegenerative diseases. Its ability to process vast volumes of patient data, coupled with its intricate algorithms, offers the potential to streamline treatment decisions and enhance patient care. However, this promising technology comes with a profound ethical consideration—the extent to which it should assume control over critical treatment decisions.

Ethical Considerations:

- *Human Oversight*: The central ethical imperative is the preservation of human oversight in healthcare decision-making. While AI, including XAI, can offer valuable insights and recommendations, healthcare providers bear ultimate responsibility for patient outcomes. They must exercise clinical judgment and accountability.
- *Patient Safety*: The foremost ethical concern is the well-being of patients. The ethical fabric of healthcare mandates that decisions, whether AI-driven or human-made, prioritize patient safety. Adverse outcomes underscore the critical importance of this ethical principle.
- *Shared Responsibility*: Ethical healthcare encourages shared responsibility between AI systems and healthcare providers. The AI should serve as a tool that augments the expertise of healthcare professionals rather than replacing it entirely. Collaboration between humans and AI is pivotal.
- *Accountability Mechanisms*: Robust mechanisms for accountability are indispensable. Ethical oversight should be in place to address instances where AI recommendations result in adverse patient outcomes. These mechanisms are crucial for learning from mistakes and continually improving AI systems.
- *Ethical Review*: Independent ethical review boards can play a crucial role in evaluating the integration of AI in healthcare settings. Their oversight ensures that ethical standards are upheld and that AI systems complement human expertise.

This scenario underscores the intricate ethical considerations surrounding the reliance on XAI systems for making treatment decisions in neurodegenerative diseases. While AI holds tremendous promise, ethical healthcare practice insists on the preservation of human judgment, shared responsibility, and robust accountability mechanisms. Ultimately, it is the harmonious partnership between human expertise and AI capabilities that ensures ethical, patient-centered care in this evolving landscape [26, 27].

4 Conclusion

As we navigate the promising yet complex intersection of eXplainable Artificial Intelligence (XAI) and neurodegenerative diseases, ethical considerations emerge as guiding beacons in our journey. The ethical landscape, defined by principles of privacy, transparency, fairness, autonomy, and accountability, resonates profoundly in this dynamic arena. In the quest to unravel the mysteries of neurodegenerative diseases, we must tread cautiously, bearing in mind that the data we harness is not just information; it's a reflection of individuals' lives. The ethical imperative of safeguarding patient data privacy, characterized by robust encryption and secure storage, respects the sanctity of this information. Furthermore, the cornerstone of informed consent fortifies the ethical foundation, ensuring that individuals have agency over the use of their data in research and clinical applications.

Transparency in AI becomes not just a technical endeavor but a moral obligation. Clear, understandable explanations of AI-driven recommendations pave the way for trust and collaboration between healthcare providers and patients. The empowerment of individuals to make informed healthcare choices is the ethical fulcrum upon which these technologies must pivot. AI, if not rigorously designed and tested, can perpetuate biases that underlie healthcare disparities. The ethical imperative is clear—to address algorithmic bias and uphold fairness. Equitable healthcare, where AI delivers consistent, unbiased recommendations across diverse demographics, is the moral compass.

In the realm of patient autonomy, AI becomes a partner, not a replacement. Ethical AI aligns with the patient's values, allowing them to retain control over their treatment decisions. It's the embodiment of ethical AI that fosters shared decision-making, recognizing that individual perspectives and choices are sacred.

Human oversight remains an ethical bulwark. Even as AI augments clinical decision-making, accountability for patient outcomes ultimately rests with healthcare providers. The ethical obligation is to establish robust accountability mechanisms to rectify AI-related errors and ensure patient safety.

The ethical path forward involves collaborative efforts across disciplines. Ethical review boards, regulatory compliance, long-term monitoring, and interdisciplinary collaborations create a harmonious ethical symphony that resonates through the journey of integrating XAI into neurodegenerative disease care. As we navigate this complex landscape, these ethical considerations are not mere constraints but guiding lights, illuminating a path where technological advancements harmonize with human values. In the ethical dance between innovation and humanity, the rhythm must always echo respect, integrity, and dignity for those whose lives are impacted by XAI in the realm of neurodegenerative diseases.

These scenarios demonstrate the importance of addressing ethical considerations when implementing XAI in the context of neurodegenerative diseases. It is essential to develop guidelines, standards, and governance structures that promote responsible and ethical AI use while maximizing the benefits of these technologies in improving patient care.

References

1. Duong, M. T., Rauschecker, A. M., & Mohan, S. (2020). Diverse applications of artificial intelligence in neuroradiology. *Neuroimaging Clinics of North America, 30*(4), 505–516. https://doi.org/10.1016/j.nic.2020.07.003. Epub 2020 Sep 17. PMID: 33039000; PMCID: PMC8530432.
2. Bhandari, M., Neupane, A., Mallik, S., Gaur, L., & Qin, H. (2023). Auguring fake face images using dual input convolution neural network. *Journal of Imaging, 9*(1), 3. https://doi.org/10.3390/jimaging9010003
3. Gaur, L., & Sahoo, B. M. (2022). Introduction to explainable AI and intelligent transportation. In *Explainable artificial intelligence for intelligent transportation systems*. Springer. https://doi.org/10.1007/978-3-031-09644-0_1
4. Ross, C. A., & Poirier, M. A. (2004). Protein aggregation and neurodegenerative disease. *Nature Medicine, 10*(Suppl), S10–S17. https://doi.org/10.1038/nm1066
5. Glass, C. K., Saijo, K., Winner, B., Marchetto, M. C., & Gage, F. H. (2010). Mechanisms underlying inflammation in neurodegeneration. *Cell, 140*, 918–934. https://doi.org/10.1016/j.cell.2010.02.016
6. Dias, V., Junn, E., & Mouradian, M. M. (2013). The role of oxidative stress in Parkinson's disease. *Journal of Parkinson's Disease, 3*, 461–491. https://doi.org/10.3233/JPD-130230
7. Shortliffe, E. H., & Buchanan, B.G. (1975). A model of inexact reasoning in medicine. *Mathematical Biosciences, 23*, 351–379. https://doi.org/10.1016/0025-5564(75)90047-4
8. Lindsay, R. K., Buchanan, B. G., Feigenbaum, E. A., & Lederberg, J. (1993). DENDRAL: A case study of the first expert system for scientific hypothesis formation. *Artificial Intelligence, 61*, 209–261 (1993). https://doi.org/10.1016/0004-3702(93)90068-M
9. Miller, R. A., Pople, H. E. J., & Myers, J. D. (1982). Internist-1, an experimental computer-based diagnostic consultant for general internal medicine. *New England Journal of Medicine, 307*, 468–476. https://doi.org/10.1056/NEJM198208193070803
10. de Dombal, F. T., Leaper, D. J., Staniland, J. R., McCann, A. P., & Horrocks, J. C. (1972). Computer-aided diagnosis of acute abdominal pain. *British Medical Journal, 2*, 9–13. https://doi.org/10.1136/bmj.2.5804.9
11. Ghose, P., Alavi, M., Tabassum, M., Ashraf Uddin, M., Biswas, M., Mahbub, K., Gaur, L., Mallik, S., & Zhao, Z. (2022). Detecting COVID-19 infection status from chest X-ray and CT scan via single transfer learning-driven approach. *Frontiers in Genetics, 13*, 980338. https://doi.org/10.3389/fgene.2022.980338
12. Gaur, L., Bhandari, M., Razdan, T., Mallik, S., & Zhao, Z. (2022). Explanation-driven deep learning model for prediction of brain tumour status using MRI image data. *Frontiers in Genetics, 13*, 822666. https://doi.org/10.3389/fgene.2022.822666
13. De Fauw, J., Ledsam, J. R., Romera-Paredes, B., Nikolov, S., Tomasev, N., Blackwell, S., Askham, H., Glorot, X., O'Donoghue, B., Visentin, D., van den Driessche, G., Lakshminarayanan, B., Meyer, C., Mackinder, F., Bouton, S., Ayoub, K., Chopra, R., King, D., Karthikesalingam, A., … Ronneberger, O. (2018). Clinically applicable deep learning for diagnosis and referral in retinal disease. *Nature Medicine, 24*, 1342–1350. https://doi.org/10.1038/s41591-018-0107-6
14. Bhandari, M., Parajuli, P., Chapagain, P., & Gaur, L. (2022). Evaluating performance of Adam optimization by proposing energy index. In K. Santosh, R. Hegadi, & U. Pal (Eds.),

Recent trends in image processing and pattern recognition. RTIP2R 2021. Communications in computer and information science (vol. 1576). Springer. https://doi.org/10.1007/978-3-031-07005-1_15
15. Raghupathi, W., & Raghupathi, V. (2014). Big data analytics in healthcare: Promise and potential. *Health Information Science and Systems, 2*, 3. https://doi.org/10.1186/2047-2501-2-3
16. Gaur, L., Bhatia, U., Jhanjhi, N. Z., et al. (2023). Medical image-based detection of COVID-19 using deep convolution neural networks. *Multimedia Systems, 29*, 1729–1738. https://doi.org/10.1007/s00530-021-00794-6
17. Alzubaidi, L., Zhang, J., Humaidi, A. J., Al-Dujaili, A., Duan, Y., Al-Shamma, O., Santamaría, J., Fadhel, M. A., Al-Amidie, M., & Farhan, L. (2021). Review of deep learning: Concepts, CNN architectures, challenges, applications, future directions. *Springer International Publishing*. https://doi.org/10.1186/s40537-021-00444-8
18. Pyrros, A., Rodriguez Fernandez, J., Borstelmann, S. M., Flanders, A., Wenzke, D., Hart, E., Horowitz, J. M., Nikolaidis, P., Willis, M., Chen, A., Cole, P., Siddiqui, N., Muzaffar, M., Muzaffar, N., McVean, J., Menchaca, M., Katsaggelos, A. K., Koyejo, S., & Galanter, W. (2022). Validation of a deep learning, value-based care model to predict mortality and comorbidities from chest radiographs in COVID-19. *PLOS Digital Health, 1*, e0000057. https://doi.org/10.1371/journal.pdig.0000057
19. Wang, L., Li, P., Hou, M., Zhang, X., Cao, X., & Li, H. (2021). Construction of a risk prediction model for Alzheimer's disease in the elderly population. *BMC Neurology, 21*, 271. https://doi.org/10.1186/s12883-021-02276-8
20. Gaur, L., Singh, G., & Agarwal, V. (2021). Leveraging artificial intelligence tools to combat the COVID-19 crisis. In P. K. Singh, G. Veselov, V. Vyatkin, A. Pljonkin, J. M. Dodero, & Y. Kumar (Eds.), *Futuristic trends in network and communication technologies. FTNCT 2020. Communications in computer and information science* (vol. 1395). Springer. https://doi.org/10.1007/978-981-16-1480-4_28
21. Sweeney, L. (2002). K-anonymity: A model for protecting privacy. *International Journal of Uncertainty, Fuzziness Knowledge-Based Systems, 10*, 557–570 (2002). https://doi.org/10.1142/S0218488502001648
22. Saeed, S., Haroon, H. B., Naqvi, M., Jhanjhi, N. Z., Ahmad, M., & Gaur, L. (2022). A systematic mapping study of low-grade tumor of brain cancer and CSF fluid detecting approaches and parameters. In N. Zaman, L. Gaur, & M. Humayun (Eds.), *Approaches and applications of deep learning in virtual medical care* (pp. 236–259). IGI Global. https://doi.org/10.4018/978-1-7998-8929-8.ch010
23. L. Gaur, U. Bhatia, & S. Bakshi. (2022). Cloud driven framework for skin cancer detection using deep CNN. In *2022 2nd international conference on innovative practices in technology and management (ICIPTM)* (pp. 460–464). https://doi.org/10.1109/ICIPTM54933.2022.9754216
24. Ghose, P., Sharmin, S., Gaur, L., & Zhao, Z. (2022). Grid-search integrated optimized support vector machine model for breast cancer detection. In *2022 IEEE international conference on bioinformatics and biomedicine (BIBM)* (pp. 2846–2852). https://doi.org/10.1109/BIBM55620.2022.9995703
25. Gaur, L., Jhanjhi, N. Z., Bakshi, S., & Gupta, P. (2022). Analyzing consequences of artificial intelligence on jobs using topic modeling and keyword extraction. In *2022 2nd international conference on innovative practices in technology and management (ICIPTM)* (pp. 435–440). https://doi.org/10.1109/ICIPTM54933.2022.9754064
26. Counts, S. E., Ikonomovic, M. D., Mercado, N., Vega, I. E., & Mufson, E. J. (2017). Biomarkers for the early detection and progression of Alzheimer's disease. *Neurotherapeutics, 14*, 35–53. https://doi.org/10.1007/s13311-016-0481-z
27. Kormas, P., & Moutzouri, A. (2020). Current psychological approaches in neurodegenerative diseases. In P. Vlamos, I. S. Kotsireas, & I. Tarnanas (Eds.), *Handbook of computational neurodegeneration* (pp. 1–29). Springer International Publishing. https://doi.org/10.1007/978-3-319-75479-6_10-1

MIX
Papier aus verantwortungsvollen Quellen
Paper from responsible sources
FSC® C105338

If you have any concerns about our products,
you can contact us on
ProductSafety@springernature.com

In case Publisher is established outside the EU,
the EU authorized representative is:
Springer Nature Customer Service Center GmbH
Europaplatz 3, 69115 Heidelberg, Germany

Printed by Libri Plureos GmbH
in Hamburg, Germany